1. Grilled salmon with steamed broccoli

Ingredients:

- 4 salmon fillets (about 4•6 oz each)
- 1 lb broccoli florets
- 2 tbsp olive oil
- 1 tbsp lemon juice
- 1 tsp garlic powder
- 1 tsp dried dill
- Salt and pepper to taste

Instructions:

1. Preheat grill or grill pan to medium•high heat.

2. In a small bowl, mix together the olive oil, lemon juice, garlic powder, and dried dill. Season with salt and pepper.

3. Brush the salmon fillets with the oil and seasoning mixture on both sides.

4. Grill the salmon for 4•6 minutes per side, or until it flakes easily with a fork.

5. While the salmon is grilling, steam the broccoli florets for 5•7 minutes until tender•crisp.

6. Serve the grilled salmon fillets with the steamed broccoli on the side.

This recipe is supportive for a fatty liver diet for women for a few reasons:

- Salmon is an excellent source of omega•3 fatty acids, which can help reduce inflammation and support liver health.

- Broccoli is high in fiber, vitamins, and antioxidants that can also benefit the liver.

- The meal is low in saturated fat and calories, which is important for managing fatty liver disease.

- The simple seasoning and cooking methods keep the dish light and easy to digest.

2. Quinoa salad with mixed greens and grilled chicken

Ingredients:

- 1 cup uncooked quinoa, rinsed
- 2 cups low•sodium chicken or vegetable broth
- 4 boneless, skinless chicken breasts
- 1 tbsp olive oil
- 1 tsp garlic powder
- Salt and pepper to taste
- 5 oz mixed greens (such as spinach, arugula, kale)
- 1 cup cherry tomatoes, halved
- 1/2 cup diced cucumber
- 2 tbsp chopped fresh parsley
- 2 tbsp lemon juice
- 1 tbsp balsamic vinegar

Instructions:

1. Cook the quinoa according to package instructions, using the broth instead of water. Allow to cool.

2. Preheat grill or grill pan to medium•high heat. Brush the chicken breasts with olive oil and season with garlic powder, salt, and pepper.

3. Grill the chicken for 5•7 minutes per side, or until cooked through. Allow to cool, then slice or shred the chicken.

4. In a large bowl, combine the cooked quinoa, mixed greens, cherry tomatoes, cucumber, and parsley.

5. Whisk together the lemon juice and balsamic vinegar. Drizzle the dressing over the salad and toss to coat. Top the salad with the grilled chicken slices.

This recipe is supportive for a fatty liver diet for women for a few reasons:

- Quinoa is a high•fiber, gluten•free grain that can help support liver health.
- Greens like spinach and kale are rich in antioxidants and vitamins that can benefit the liver.
- Grilled chicken is a lean protein source that is easy to digest.
- The salad is low in saturated fat and calories, which is important for managing fatty liver disease.
- The lemon juice and balsamic vinegar provide a light, flavorful dressing without added sugars or oils.

Welcome to the ***"Fatty Liver Diet Cookbook for Women: 110+ Wholesome Meals to Nurture Your Liver and Well-being."*** This book is your comprehensive guide to understanding and managing fatty liver disease through delicious, nutritious, and easy-to-make recipes tailored specifically for women.

Fatty liver disease, also known as hepatic steatosis, is a condition characterized by excess fat accumulation in the liver. While it can affect anyone, women often face unique challenges due to hormonal changes, metabolic differences, and lifestyle factors. This cookbook aims to provide you with practical and enjoyable solutions to support your liver health, improve your overall well-being, and help you reclaim your vitality.

Understanding Fatty Liver Disease

Before diving into the recipes, it's important to understand the basics of fatty liver disease. This condition can be influenced by various factors such as diet, genetics, lifestyle, and underlying health conditions. Left unmanaged, fatty liver disease can lead to more serious liver issues, including inflammation, fibrosis, and cirrhosis. However, the good news is that dietary and lifestyle changes can significantly improve liver health and even reverse the progression of the disease.

The Power of Nutrition

The foundation of managing and reversing fatty liver disease lies in a balanced, nutrient-rich diet. This cookbook focuses on providing wholesome meals that are low in unhealthy fats and sugars, yet rich in fiber, antioxidants, and essential nutrients. By incorporating these recipes into your daily routine, you can help reduce liver fat, decrease inflammation, and promote liver regeneration.

Why This Cookbook?

This cookbook is designed with women in mind. Women's nutritional needs can vary based on life stages, hormonal fluctuations, and metabolic changes. The recipes in this book are crafted to not only support liver health but also cater to these unique requirements. Whether you are a busy professional, a mom juggling multiple responsibilities, or someone looking to improve their health, this cookbook offers practical, flavorful, and health-boosting recipes that fit seamlessly into your lifestyle.

What You'll Find Inside

- ***110+ Wholesome Recipes:*** From breakfast to dinner, snacks to desserts, each recipe is thoughtfully created to nourish your liver and delight your taste buds.

- ***Nutritional Guidance:*** Learn about the key nutrients and food groups that play a vital role in liver health, and how to incorporate them into your diet.

- ***Meal Planning Tips:*** Practical advice on meal prepping, grocery shopping, and creating balanced meal plans that support your liver health.

- ***Lifestyle Recommendations:*** Beyond diet, discover lifestyle changes that can enhance your overall well-being and complement your dietary efforts.

A Journey to Better Health

Embarking on a fatty liver diet is more than just changing what you eat; it's about adopting a healthier, more mindful way of living. This cookbook is your companion on this journey, providing you with the tools, knowledge, and delicious recipes to make lasting, positive changes.

Thank you for choosing ***"Fatty Liver Diet Cookbook for Women."*** Here's to nurturing your liver, enhancing your well-being, and enjoying every step of the way with wholesome, satisfying meals.

Warm wishes,

3. Baked sweet potatoes with a side of green beans

Ingredients:
- 4 medium sweet potatoes, scrubbed clean
- 1 lb fresh green beans, trimmed
- 2 tbsp olive oil
- 2 cloves garlic, minced
- 1 tsp dried thyme
- Salt and pepper to taste

Instructions:

1. Preheat the oven to 400°F. Pierce the sweet potatoes a few times with a fork and place them directly on the oven rack. Bake for 45•60 minutes, until tender when pierced with a fork.

2. While the sweet potatoes are baking, prepare the green beans. In a large skillet, heat the olive oil over medium heat. Add the minced garlic and sauté for 1 minute until fragrant.

3. Add the green beans to the skillet and sauté for 5•7 minutes, stirring occasionally, until the beans are tender•crisp. Season with the dried thyme, salt, and pepper.

4. Once the sweet potatoes are cooked through, remove them from the oven and let cool slightly. Slice each potato in half lengthwise.

5. Serve the baked sweet potato halves with the sautéed green beans on the side.

This recipe is supportive for a fatty liver diet for women for a few reasons:

- Sweet potatoes are a nutrient•dense carbohydrate source that is high in fiber, vitamins, and antioxidants that can benefit liver health.

- Green beans are a low•calorie, high•fiber vegetable that can also support liver function.

- The simple preparation methods, without added fats or sugars, keep the dish light and easy to digest.

- This meal is low in saturated fat and calories, which is important for managing fatty liver disease.

4. Turkey chili with kidney beans and vegetables

Ingredients:

- 1 lb ground turkey
- 1 onion, diced
- 3 cloves garlic, minced
- 2 bell peppers, diced
- 1 tsp ground cumin
- 1 tsp dried oregano
- Salt and pepper to taste

- 2 carrots, peeled and diced
- 2 celery stalks, diced
- 1 (15 oz) can kidney beans, rinsed and drained
- 1 (15 oz) can diced tomatoes
- 2 cups low•sodium chicken or vegetable broth
- 2 tbsp chili powder

Instructions:

1. In a large pot or Dutch oven, cook the ground turkey over medium•high heat, breaking it up with a wooden spoon, until browned and cooked through, about 5•7 minutes. Drain any excess fat.

2. Add the diced onion, garlic, bell peppers, carrots, and celery to the pot. Sauté for 5•7 minutes, until the vegetables are tender.

3. Stir in the kidney beans, diced tomatoes, broth, chili powder, cumin, and oregano. Season with salt and pepper to taste.

4. Bring the chili to a simmer and let it cook for 20•30 minutes, stirring occasionally, until the flavors have melded and the chili has thickened.

5. Serve the turkey chili hot, garnished with any desired toppings like avocado, cilantro, or low•fat sour cream.

This recipe is supportive for a fatty liver diet for women for a few reasons:

• Ground turkey is a lean protein source that is easy to digest.

• Kidney beans are high in fiber and protein, which can help support liver health.

• The vegetables like bell peppers, carrots, and celery provide a variety of vitamins, minerals, and antioxidants.

• The chili is low in saturated fat and calories, which is important for managing fatty liver disease. The spices like chili powder and cumin add flavor without added sugars or oils.

5. Roasted vegetables with olive oil

Ingredients:

• 2 bell peppers, cut into 1•inch pieces
• 2 zucchini, cut into 1•inch pieces
• 3 carrots, peeled and cut into 1•inch pieces
• 1 red onion, cut into 1•inch pieces
• 2 tbsp olive oil
• 1 tsp dried thyme
• 1 tsp dried oregano
• Salt and pepper to taste

Instructions:

1. Preheat the oven to 400°F. Line a large baking sheet with parchment paper.

2. In a large bowl, toss the chopped bell peppers, zucchini, carrots, and red onion with the olive oil, dried thyme, dried oregano, salt, and pepper until the vegetables are evenly coated.

3. Spread the seasoned vegetables in a single layer on the prepared baking sheet.

4. Roast the vegetables for 25•30 minutes, stirring halfway, until they are tender and lightly browned.

5. Serve the roasted vegetables warm, as a side dish or mixed into other dishes.

This recipe is supportive for a fatty liver diet for women for a few reasons:

• The vegetables like bell peppers, zucchini, and carrots are high in fiber, vitamins, and antioxidants that can benefit liver health.

• Olive oil is a healthy monounsaturated fat that can help reduce inflammation and support liver function.

• The simple roasting method without added sugars or heavy sauces keeps the dish light and easy to digest.

• This meal is low in saturated fat and calories, which is important for managing fatty liver disease.

The combination of nutrient•dense vegetables and heart•healthy olive oil makes this a great option for a fatty liver diet.

6. Stir fried tofu with mixed vegetables

Ingredients:

- 1 red bell pepper, sliced
- 1 cup broccoli florets
- 1 cup sliced mushrooms
- 1 cup snow peas or snap peas
- 2 cups baby spinach
- Salt and pepper to taste

- 1 block (14 oz) extra•firm tofu, pressed and cubed
- 2 tbsp low•sodium soy sauce or tamari
- 1 tbsp rice vinegar
- 1 tsp sesame oil
- 1 tbsp olive oil
- 3 cloves garlic, minced
- 1 inch fresh ginger, peeled and grated

Instructions:

1. In a small bowl, whisk together the soy sauce, rice vinegar, and sesame oil. Set aside.

2. Heat the olive oil in a large skillet or wok over medium•high heat. Add the cubed tofu and sauté for 5•7 minutes, turning occasionally, until lightly browned on all sides. Transfer the tofu to a plate.

3. In the same skillet, add the minced garlic and grated ginger. Sauté for 1 minute until fragrant.

4. Add the sliced bell pepper, broccoli, mushrooms, and snow peas. Stir•fry for 5•7 minutes, until the vegetables are tender•crisp.

5. Return the sautéed tofu to the skillet and pour in the soy sauce mixture. Toss everything together and cook for 2•3 minutes, until the sauce has thickened slightly.

6. Remove from heat and stir in the baby spinach. Season with salt and pepper to taste. Serve the stir•fried tofu and vegetables immediately, over brown rice or quinoa if desired.

This recipe is supportive for a fatty liver diet for women for a few reasons:

- Tofu is a plant•based protein that is easy to digest and low in saturated fat.

- The mixed vegetables provide a variety of vitamins, minerals, and antioxidants that can benefit liver health.

- The stir•fry method uses minimal oil, keeping the dish light and low in calories.

- The soy sauce and rice vinegar add flavor without added sugars.

7. Lentil soup with spinach and carrots

Ingredients:

• 1 cup dry brown or green lentils, rinsed
• 4 cups low•sodium vegetable or chicken broth
• 2 carrots, peeled and diced
• 1 onion, diced
• 3 cloves garlic, minced
• 2 tsp ground cumin
• 1 tsp dried thyme
• 1/4 tsp cayenne pepper (optional)
• 4 cups fresh spinach, chopped
• Salt and pepper to taste
• Lemon wedges for serving (optional)

Instructions:

1. In a large pot, combine the rinsed lentils and broth. Bring to a boil over high heat.

2. Once boiling, reduce heat to medium•low and let the lentils simmer for 15•20 minutes, until tender.

3. Add the diced carrots, onion, and garlic to the pot. Stir in the cumin, thyme, and cayenne (if using).

4. Continue simmering for 10•15 minutes, until the vegetables are tender.

5. Stir in the chopped spinach and cook for 2•3 minutes more, until the spinach is wilted.

6. Season the soup with salt and pepper to taste. Serve the lentil soup hot, with a squeeze of lemon juice over the top if desired.

This recipe is supportive for a fatty liver diet for women for a few reasons:

• Lentils are a high•fiber, plant•based protein that can help support liver health.
• Spinach is packed with vitamins, minerals, and antioxidants that are beneficial for the liver.
• Carrots provide beta•carotene and other nutrients that may help protect the liver.
• The simple, vegetable•based soup is low in saturated fat and calories, which is important for managing fatty liver disease.
• The spices like cumin and thyme add flavor without added sugars or oils.

8. Baked chicken breast with roasted asparagus

Ingredients:

• 4 boneless, skinless chicken breasts
• 1 tbsp olive oil
• 1 tsp garlic powder
• 1 tsp dried oregano
• Salt and pepper to taste
• 1 lb asparagus, trimmed
• 1 tbsp lemon juice

Instructions:

1. Preheat the oven to 400°F. Line a baking sheet with parchment paper.

2. Place the chicken breasts on the prepared baking sheet. Drizzle with the olive oil and sprinkle with the garlic powder, dried oregano, salt, and pepper. Rub the seasoning all over the chicken.

3. Arrange the trimmed asparagus spears around the chicken on the baking sheet.

4. Bake for 20•25 minutes, or until the chicken is cooked through (internal temperature reaches 165°F) and the asparagus is tender•crisp.

5. Remove the baked chicken and asparagus from the oven. Drizzle the asparagus with the lemon juice.

6. Serve the baked chicken breast with the roasted asparagus on the side.

This recipe is supportive for a fatty liver diet for women for a few reasons:

• Chicken breast is a lean protein source that is easy to digest.

• Asparagus is high in fiber, vitamins, and antioxidants that can benefit liver health.

• The simple baking method without added sauces or heavy seasonings keeps the dish light and low in calories.

• The lemon juice provides a bright, flavorful accent without added sugars or oils.

• This meal is low in saturated fat and calories, which is important for managing fatty liver disease.

9. Whole grain pasta with marinara sauce and lean ground turkey

Ingredients:

• 8 oz whole grain pasta (such as whole wheat or chickpea pasta)
• 1 lb lean ground turkey
• 1 onion, diced
• 3 cloves garlic, minced
• 1 (28 oz) can crushed tomatoes
• 2 tbsp tomato paste
• 1 tsp dried oregano
• 1 tsp dried basil
• 1/4 tsp red pepper flakes (optional)
• Salt and pepper to taste
• Grated Parmesan cheese for serving (optional)

Instructions:

1. Bring a large pot of salted water to a boil. Cook the whole grain pasta according to package instructions until al dente. Drain and set aside.

2. In a large skillet or Dutch oven, cook the lean ground turkey over medium•high heat, breaking it up with a wooden spoon, until browned and cooked through, about 5•7 minutes. Drain any excess fat.

3. Add the diced onion and minced garlic to the skillet. Sauté for 2•3 minutes until the onion is translucent.

4. Stir in the crushed tomatoes, tomato paste, dried oregano, dried basil, and red pepper flakes (if using). Season with salt and pepper to taste.

5. Reduce the heat to medium•low and let the marinara sauce simmer for 10•15 minutes, stirring occasionally, to allow the flavors to meld.

6. Add the cooked whole grain pasta to the skillet and toss to coat with the marinara sauce.

7. Serve the pasta and turkey marinara warm, with grated Parmesan cheese on top if desired.

This recipe is supportive for a fatty liver diet for women for a few reasons:

• Whole grain pasta is a complex carbohydrate that is high in fiber, which can help support liver health.

10. Steamed fish with ginger and soy sauce

Ingredients:

- 4 (4•6 oz) white fish fillets (such as cod, tilapia, or halibut)
- 2 tbsp low•sodium soy sauce
- 1 tbsp rice vinegar
- 1 tbsp freshly grated ginger
- 2 tsp sesame oil
- 2 green onions, thinly sliced
- Chopped cilantro for garnish (optional)

Instructions:

1. Set up a steamer basket in a large pot with about 1 inch of water in the bottom. Bring the water to a boil over high heat.

2. In a small bowl, whisk together the soy sauce, rice vinegar, grated ginger, and sesame oil.

3. Place the fish fillets in the steamer basket. Pour the soy sauce mixture over the top of the fish.

4. Cover the pot and steam the fish for 8•10 minutes, or until it flakes easily with a fork.

5. Transfer the steamed fish to a serving plate. Drizzle any remaining sauce from the steamer over the top.

6. Garnish the fish with the sliced green onions and chopped cilantro (if using). Serve the steamed fish immediately, with steamed vegetables or brown rice on the side.

This recipe is supportive for a fatty liver diet for women for a few reasons:

- Fish, especially white fish like cod or tilapia, is a lean protein source that is easy to digest.

- Ginger and soy sauce provide flavor without added sugars or oils.

- Steaming the fish preserves its nutrients and keeps the dish light and low in calories.

- The green onions and optional cilantro add freshness and antioxidants.

- This meal is low in saturated fat and high in protein, which is important for managing fatty liver disease.

11. Vegetable omelet with whole grain toast

Ingredients:

- 3 large eggs
- 2 tbsp low•fat milk
- 1 tsp olive oil
- 1/2 cup diced bell peppers
- 1/2 cup sliced mushrooms
- 1/4 cup diced onion
- 2 cups baby spinach leaves
- 2 tbsp grated low•fat cheddar cheese (optional)
- Salt and pepper to taste
- 2 slices whole grain toast

Instructions:

1. In a small bowl, whisk together the eggs and milk. Season with a pinch of salt and pepper.

2. Heat the olive oil in a nonstick skillet over medium heat. Add the diced bell peppers, mushrooms, and onion. Sauté for 3•4 minutes until the vegetables are tender.

3. Pour the egg mixture into the skillet and let it sit for 30 seconds to 1 minute, until the edges start to set.

4. Using a spatula, gently push the cooked egg towards the center, tilting the pan to allow the uncooked egg to flow to the edges. Continue this process until the omelet is mostly set, about 2•3 minutes.

5. Sprinkle the baby spinach leaves over the top of the omelet and let them wilt for 1 minute. If using, sprinkle the grated cheddar cheese over the top of the omelet.

7. Fold the omelet in half and slide it onto a plate. Serve the vegetable omelet immediately, with 2 slices of whole grain toast on the side.

This recipe is supportive for a fatty liver diet for women for a few reasons:

- Eggs are a high•quality protein source that is easy to digest. The vegetables like bell peppers, mushrooms, onions, and spinach provide a variety of vitamins, minerals, and antioxidants that can benefit liver health.

- Whole grain toast is a complex carbohydrate that is high in fiber.

- The dish is low in saturated fat and calories, which is important for managing fatty liver disease.

- The simple preparation method without added oils or heavy sauces keeps the meal light and nutritious.

12. Brown rice stir fry with shrimp and vegetables

Ingredients:

- 1 cup uncooked brown rice
- 1 lb raw shrimp, peeled and deveined
- 2 tbsp low•sodium soy sauce or tamari
- 1 tbsp rice vinegar
- 1 tsp sesame oil
- 1 tbsp olive oil
- 1 inch fresh ginger, peeled and grated
- 1 red bell pepper, sliced
- 1 cup broccoli florets
- 1 cup sliced mushrooms
- 3 cloves garlic, minced
- 2 cups baby spinach
- Salt and pepper to taste
- Chopped green onions for garnish (optional)

Instructions:

1. Cook the brown rice according to package instructions. Set aside.

2. In a small bowl, whisk together the soy sauce, rice vinegar, and sesame oil. Set aside.

3. Heat the olive oil in a large skillet or wok over medium•high heat. Add the shrimp and sauté for 2•3 minutes, until partially cooked. Transfer the shrimp to a plate.

4. In the same skillet, add the minced garlic and grated ginger. Sauté for 1 minute until fragrant.

5. Add the sliced bell pepper, broccoli florets, and mushrooms to the skillet. Stir•fry for 5•7 minutes, until the vegetables are tender•crisp.

6. Return the partially cooked shrimp to the skillet. Pour in the soy sauce mixture and toss everything together.

7. Add the cooked brown rice and baby spinach to the skillet. Stir•fry for 2•3 minutes, until the spinach is wilted and the rice is heated through.

8. Season the stir•fry with salt and pepper to taste. Serve the brown rice stir•fry hot, garnished with chopped green onions if desired.

This recipe is supportive for a fatty liver diet for women for a few reasons:

• Brown rice is a whole grain that is high in fiber, which can help support liver health. Shrimp is a lean protein source that is easy to digest.

• The mixed vegetables like bell peppers, broccoli, and spinach provide a variety of vitamins, minerals, and antioxidants.

• The stir•fry method uses minimal oil, keeping the dish light and low in calories. The soy sauce and rice vinegar add flavor without added sugars.

13. Greek yogurt parfait with berries and almonds

Ingredients:
• 2 cups plain Greek yogurt
• 1 cup mixed berries (such as blueberries, raspberries, and/or strawberries)
• 1/4 cup sliced or chopped almonds
• 1 tbsp honey (optional)

Instructions:

1. In a parfait glass or bowl, layer half of the Greek yogurt on the bottom.

2. Top the yogurt with half of the mixed berries.

3. Sprinkle half of the sliced almonds over the berries.

4. Repeat the layers, ending with the remaining yogurt, berries, and almonds.

5. If desired, drizzle the honey over the top of the parfait.

6. Serve the Greek yogurt parfait chilled.

This recipe is supportive for a fatty liver diet for women for a few reasons:

• Greek yogurt is a high•protein, low•fat dairy product that can help support liver health.

• Berries are rich in antioxidants and fiber, which are beneficial for the liver.

• Almonds are a source of healthy fats, fiber, and vitamins that may help protect the liver.

• The parfait is low in added sugars, as the honey is optional.

• This dessert•like dish is light, refreshing, and easy to digest.

14. Spinach salad with grilled shrimp and avocado

Ingredients:

- 5 oz baby spinach leaves
- 1 lb raw shrimp, peeled and deveined
- 1 tbsp olive oil
- 1 tsp lemon juice
- 1 tsp dried oregano
- Salt and pepper to taste
- 1 avocado, diced
- 2 tbsp balsamic vinaigrette (or use a lemon•based dressing)

Instructions:

1. Preheat grill or grill pan to medium•high heat.

2. In a small bowl, toss the shrimp with the olive oil, lemon juice, dried oregano, salt, and pepper.

3. Grill the seasoned shrimp for 2•3 minutes per side, until opaque and cooked through. Remove from heat and set aside.

4. In a large salad bowl, arrange the baby spinach leaves.

5. Top the spinach with the grilled shrimp and diced avocado.

6. Drizzle the balsamic vinaigrette (or lemon•based dressing) over the salad.

7. Toss the salad gently to coat the ingredients with the dressing.

8. Serve the spinach salad with grilled shrimp and avocado immediately.

This recipe is supportive for a fatty liver diet for women for a few reasons:

- Spinach is a nutrient•dense green that is high in vitamins, minerals, and antioxidants to support liver health.

- Shrimp is a lean protein source that is easy to digest.

- Avocado provides healthy monounsaturated fats that can help reduce inflammation.

- The simple grilled shrimp and light dressing keep the dish low in calories and saturated fat. This salad is well•balanced with protein, healthy fats, and fiber•rich vegetables.

15. Baked cod with lemon and herbs, served with quinoa

Ingredients:

• 4 (4•6 oz) cod fillets
• 2 tbsp olive oil
• 2 tbsp lemon juice
• 1 tsp dried parsley
• 1 tsp dried dill
• 1/2 tsp garlic powder
• Salt and pepper to taste
• 1 cup uncooked quinoa, rinsed
• 2 cups low•sodium vegetable or chicken broth

Instructions:

1. Preheat the oven to 400°F. Line a baking sheet with parchment paper.

2. In a small bowl, whisk together the olive oil, lemon juice, dried parsley, dried dill, and garlic powder. Season with salt and pepper.

3. Place the cod fillets on the prepared baking sheet. Brush the tops of the cod with the lemon•herb mixture.

4. Bake the cod for 12•15 minutes, or until it flakes easily with a fork.

5. While the cod is baking, cook the quinoa. In a medium saucepan, combine the rinsed quinoa and broth. Bring to a boil over high heat.

6. Once boiling, reduce the heat to low, cover the saucepan, and simmer for 15•20 minutes, until the quinoa is tender and the liquid is absorbed.

7. Fluff the cooked quinoa with a fork. Serve the baked cod fillets warm, over a bed of the cooked quinoa.

This recipe is supportive for a fatty liver diet for women for a few reasons:

• Cod is a lean, white fish that is high in protein and low in mercury, making it a great choice for liver health. The lemon and herb seasoning adds flavor without added sugars or oils.

• Quinoa is a high•fiber, gluten•free grain that can help support liver function.

• This meal is low in saturated fat and calories, which is important for managing fatty liver disease.

16. Veggie burger on a whole grain bun with a side salad

Ingredients:

• 4 veggie burger patties (look for ones made with beans, lentils, or vegetables)
• 4 whole grain hamburger buns
• 1 head of romaine lettuce, chopped
• 1 cup cherry tomatoes, halved
• 1/2 cucumber, sliced
• 1/4 red onion, thinly sliced
• 2 tbsp balsamic vinaigrette
• Salt and pepper to taste

Instructions:

1. Preheat the oven or grill to the temperature recommended on the veggie burger packaging.

2. Cook the veggie burger patties according to the package instructions, until heated through and lightly browned.

3. While the veggie burgers are cooking, prepare the side salad. In a large bowl, combine the chopped romaine lettuce, cherry tomatoes, cucumber slices, and red onion slices.

4. Drizzle the balsamic vinaigrette over the salad and toss gently to coat. Season with salt and pepper to taste.

5. Place the cooked veggie burger patties on the whole grain buns. Serve the veggie burgers immediately, with the side salad on the plate.

This recipe is supportive for a fatty liver diet for women for a few reasons:

• Veggie burgers made with beans, lentils, or vegetables are a great source of plant-based protein and fiber, which can benefit liver health.

• Whole grain buns provide complex carbohydrates and additional fiber.

• The side salad with romaine lettuce, tomatoes, cucumber, and onion is packed with vitamins, minerals, and antioxidants.

• The balsamic vinaigrette dressing adds flavor without added sugars or oils. This meal is low in saturated fat and calories, which is important for managing fatty liver disease.

17. Chicken and vegetable skewers grilled with a light marinade

Ingredients:

• 1 lb boneless, skinless chicken breasts, cut into 1·inch cubes
• 1 red bell pepper, cut into 1·inch pieces
• 1 zucchini, cut into 1·inch pieces
• 1 red onion, cut into 1·inch pieces
• 8 oz mushrooms, halved
• 2 tbsp olive oil
• 2 tbsp lemon juice
• 1 tsp dried oregano
• 1 tsp garlic powder
• Salt and pepper to taste
• Wooden or metal skewers

Instructions:

1. In a large bowl, whisk together the olive oil, lemon juice, dried oregano, garlic powder, salt, and pepper.

2. Add the cubed chicken, bell pepper, zucchini, onion, and mushrooms to the bowl. Toss to coat the ingredients evenly with the marinade.

3. Thread the marinated chicken and vegetables onto the skewers, alternating the ingredients. Preheat the grill or grill pan to medium·high heat.

4. Grill the skewers for 12·15 minutes, turning occasionally, until the chicken is cooked through and the vegetables are tender. Serve the grilled chicken and vegetable skewers immediately.

This recipe is supportive for a fatty liver diet for women for a few reasons:

• Chicken breast is a lean protein source that is easy to digest. The mixed vegetables like bell peppers, zucchini, onions, and mushrooms provide a variety of vitamins, minerals, and antioxidants that can benefit liver health.

• The simple marinade with lemon juice, olive oil, and herbs adds flavor without added sugars or heavy sauces.

• Grilling the skewers keeps the dish light and low in calories. This meal is well·balanced with protein, vegetables, and healthy fats, making it a great option for a fatty liver diet.

18. Turkey meatballs with whole wheat spaghetti

Ingredients:

- 1 lb ground turkey
- 1/2 cup whole wheat breadcrumbs
- 1 egg
- 2 tbsp grated Parmesan cheese
- 2 cloves garlic, minced
- 1 tsp dried oregano
- 1/2 tsp salt
- 1/4 tsp black pepper
- 8 oz whole wheat spaghetti
- 1 (24 oz) jar low•sodium marinara sauce
- 2 tbsp chopped fresh basil (optional)

Instructions:

1. Preheat the oven to 400°F. Line a baking sheet with parchment paper.

2. In a large bowl, combine the ground turkey, breadcrumbs, egg, Parmesan, garlic, oregano, salt, and pepper. Mix until well incorporated.

3. Roll the turkey mixture into 1•inch meatballs and place them on the prepared baking sheet.

4. Bake the meatballs for 18•20 minutes, until cooked through.

5. While the meatballs are baking, cook the whole wheat spaghetti according to package instructions. Drain and set aside. In a large saucepan, heat the marinara sauce over medium heat until warmed through.

6. Add the cooked turkey meatballs to the marinara sauce and gently toss to coat. Serve the turkey meatballs and marinara sauce over the cooked whole wheat spaghetti. Garnish with chopped fresh basil, if desired.

This recipe is supportive for a fatty liver diet for women for a few reasons:

- Ground turkey is a lean protein source that is easy to digest.

- Whole wheat spaghetti is a complex carbohydrate that is high in fiber, which can benefit liver health. The marinara sauce is a tomato•based sauce that is rich in antioxidants.

- The simple preparation method without added oils or heavy creams keeps the dish light and low in calories.

19. Eggplant parmesan with a side of mixed greens

Ingredients:

Eggplant Parmesan:
• 1 medium eggplant, sliced into 1/2•inch rounds
• 1 cup whole wheat breadcrumbs
• 1/2 cup grated Parmesan cheese
• 1 tsp dried oregano
• 1/2 tsp garlic powder
• 1/4 tsp salt
• 2 eggs, beaten
• 1 (24 oz) jar low•sodium marinara sauce
• 1 cup shredded part•skim mozzarella cheese

Mixed Greens Salad:
• 5 oz mixed greens (such as spinach, arugula, and kale)
• 1 cup cherry tomatoes, halved
• 1/4 cup sliced cucumber
• 2 tbsp balsamic vinaigrette

Instructions:

Eggplant Parmesan:

1. Preheat the oven to 400°F. Line a baking sheet with parchment paper.

2. In a shallow bowl, combine the breadcrumbs, Parmesan, oregano, garlic powder, and salt.

3. Dip the eggplant slices in the beaten eggs, then coat them in the breadcrumb mixture, pressing to adhere.

4. Arrange the breaded eggplant slices on the prepared baking sheet. Bake for 20•25 minutes, flipping halfway, until golden brown.

5. Spread a thin layer of marinara sauce in the bottom of a baking dish. Arrange the baked eggplant slices in a single layer. Top with the remaining marinara sauce and shredded mozzarella. Bake for an additional 15•20 minutes, until the cheese is melted and bubbly.

Mixed Greens Salad:

1. In a large bowl, combine the mixed greens, cherry tomatoes, and sliced cucumber.

2. Drizzle the balsamic vinaigrette over the salad and toss to coat.

20. Baked chicken thighs with roasted Brussels sprouts

Ingredients:

- 6 bone•in, skin•on chicken thighs
- 1 tbsp olive oil
- 1 tsp garlic powder
- 1 tsp dried thyme
- 1/2 tsp salt
- 1/4 tsp black pepper
- 1 lb Brussels sprouts, trimmed and halved
- 2 tbsp olive oil
- 1 tbsp lemon juice
- 1 tsp Dijon mustard
- 1 clove garlic, minced
- Salt and pepper to taste

Instructions:

1. Preheat the oven to 400°F. Line a large baking sheet with parchment paper.

2. In a small bowl, mix together the 1 tbsp olive oil, garlic powder, dried thyme, 1/2 tsp salt, and 1/4 tsp black pepper. Rub this seasoning mixture all over the chicken thighs.

3. Arrange the seasoned chicken thighs on one side of the prepared baking sheet.

4. In a medium bowl, toss the trimmed and halved Brussels sprouts with the 2 tbsp olive oil, lemon juice, Dijon mustard, minced garlic, and a pinch of salt and pepper.

5. Spread the seasoned Brussels sprouts on the other side of the baking sheet, in a single layer.

6. Bake the chicken and Brussels sprouts for 35•40 minutes, or until the chicken is cooked through (internal temperature reaches 165°F) and the Brussels sprouts are tender and lightly browned.

7. Serve the baked chicken thighs with the roasted Brussels sprouts.

The combination of baked chicken and roasted Brussels sprouts creates a nutritious and liver•friendly meal.

21. Quinoa stuffed bell peppers

Ingredients:

• 4 medium bell peppers (any color)
• 1 cup uncooked quinoa, rinsed
• 2 cups low•sodium vegetable or chicken broth
• 1 (15 oz) can black beans, rinsed and drained
• 1 cup diced tomatoes
• 1/2 cup diced onion
• 2 cloves garlic, minced
• 1 tsp ground cumin
• 1 tsp dried oregano
• 1/4 tsp cayenne pepper (optional)
• Salt and pepper to taste
• 1/2 cup shredded low•fat cheddar cheese (optional)

Instructions:

1. Preheat the oven to 375°F. Cut the tops off the bell peppers and remove the seeds and membranes. Place the peppers in a baking dish.

2. In a medium saucepan, combine the rinsed quinoa and broth. Bring to a boil, then reduce heat to low, cover, and simmer for 15•20 minutes, until the quinoa is tender and the liquid is absorbed.

3. In a large bowl, mix the cooked quinoa, black beans, diced tomatoes, onion, garlic, cumin, oregano, and cayenne (if using). Season with salt and pepper to taste.

4. Stuff the quinoa mixture into the hollowed•out bell peppers, packing it in tightly.

5. If using the shredded cheddar cheese, sprinkle it evenly over the tops of the stuffed peppers.

6. Bake the stuffed peppers for 25•30 minutes, until the peppers are tender and the filling is hot.

7. Serve the quinoa stuffed bell peppers warm.

The combination of quinoa, beans, and vegetables in a stuffed pepper makes for a nourishing and liver•friendly meal.

22. Grilled shrimp tacos
with avocado and cabbage slaw

Ingredients:

- 1 lb raw shrimp, peeled and deveined
- 1 tbsp olive oil
- 1 tsp chili powder
- 1/2 tsp cumin
- 1/4 tsp garlic powder
- Salt and pepper to taste
- 8•10 small corn or whole wheat tortillas
- 1 avocado, diced
- 2 cups shredded purple cabbage
- 1/4 cup diced red onion
- 2 tbsp chopped cilantro
- 2 tbsp lime juice
- 1 tbsp olive oil
- Salt and pepper to taste

Instructions:

1. Preheat grill or grill pan to medium•high heat.

2. In a medium bowl, toss the shrimp with the 1 tbsp olive oil, chili powder, cumin, garlic powder, salt, and pepper.

3. Grill the seasoned shrimp for 2•3 minutes per side, until opaque and cooked through. Remove from heat and set aside.

4. In a separate bowl, combine the shredded purple cabbage, diced red onion, chopped cilantro, lime juice, 1 tbsp olive oil, salt, and pepper. Toss to coat.

5. To assemble the tacos, place a few pieces of grilled shrimp in each tortilla. Top with the cabbage slaw and diced avocado.

6. Serve the grilled shrimp tacos immediately.

The combination of grilled shrimp, avocado, and crunchy cabbage slaw makes for a flavorful and liver•friendly taco dish.

23. Turkey and vegetable stir fry with brown rice

Ingredients:

- 1 cup uncooked brown rice
- 1 lb ground turkey
- 1 tbsp sesame oil
- 2 cloves garlic, minced
- 1 inch fresh ginger, peeled and grated
- 1 red bell pepper, sliced
- 1 cup broccoli florets
- 1 cup sliced mushrooms
- 2 cups baby spinach
- 2 tbsp low•sodium soy sauce or tamari
- 1 tbsp rice vinegar
- 1 tsp sesame seeds (optional)
- Salt and pepper to taste

Instructions:

1. Cook the brown rice according to package instructions. Set aside.

2. In a large skillet or wok, heat the sesame oil over medium•high heat. Add the ground turkey and cook, breaking it up with a wooden spoon, until browned and cooked through, about 5•7 minutes.

3. Add the minced garlic and grated ginger to the skillet. Sauté for 1 minute until fragrant.

4. Stir in the sliced bell pepper, broccoli florets, and mushrooms. Sauté for 5•7 minutes, until the vegetables are tender•crisp.

5. Add the baby spinach to the skillet and cook for 2•3 minutes, until the spinach is wilted.

6. Pour in the soy sauce and rice vinegar. Toss everything together until well combined.

7. Serve the turkey and vegetable stir•fry over the cooked brown rice. Sprinkle with sesame seeds, if desired.

This balanced and nutrient•dense turkey and vegetable stir•fry makes a great option for a fatty liver diet.

24. Spinach and mushroom frittata

Ingredients:

- 8 large eggs
- 1/4 cup unsweetened almond milk
- 1/4 tsp salt
- 1/4 tsp black pepper
- 1 tbsp olive oil
- 8 oz sliced mushrooms
- 2 cups fresh spinach, chopped
- 1/4 cup crumbled feta cheese (optional)

Instructions:

1. Preheat the oven to 375°F. Grease a 9•inch oven•safe skillet or pie dish with nonstick cooking spray.

2. In a large bowl, whisk together the eggs, almond milk, salt, and pepper until well combined.

3. In the greased skillet or pie dish, heat the olive oil over medium heat. Add the sliced mushrooms and sauté for 3•4 minutes, until softened.

4. Add the chopped spinach to the skillet and cook for 1•2 minutes, until the spinach is wilted.

5. Pour the egg mixture over the mushrooms and spinach. Sprinkle the crumbled feta cheese over the top, if using.

6. Transfer the skillet or pie dish to the preheated oven and bake for 18•22 minutes, until the center of the frittata is set.

7. Remove the frittata from the oven and let it cool for 5 minutes before slicing and serving.

This spinach and mushroom frittata is a great option for a nutritious and liver•friendly breakfast or brunch.

25. Baked tilapia with a mango salsa

Ingredients:

• 4 tilapia fillets
• 1 tbsp olive oil
• 1 tsp paprika
• Salt and pepper to taste

For the Mango Salsa:
• 1 ripe mango, diced
• 1/2 red onion, finely chopped
• 1 jalapeño, seeded and finely chopped
• 1 tbsp fresh lime juice
• 2 tbsp chopped fresh cilantro
• Salt and pepper to taste

Instructions:

1. Preheat oven to 400°F. Line a baking sheet with parchment paper.

2. Place the tilapia fillets on the prepared baking sheet. Brush the fillets with olive oil and sprinkle with paprika, salt, and pepper.

3. Bake for 12•15 minutes, until the fish flakes easily with a fork.

4. Meanwhile, make the mango salsa. In a medium bowl, combine the diced mango, red onion, jalapeño, lime juice, cilantro, salt, and pepper. Stir to mix well.

5. Serve the baked tilapia warm, topped with the fresh mango salsa.

This dish is a great option for a fatty liver diet as tilapia is a lean, low•fat protein and the mango salsa provides healthy fats, fiber, and antioxidants. The combination of the baked fish and vibrant salsa makes for a delicious and nutritious meal.

26. Lentil salad with mixed vegetables and a balsamic vinaigrette

Ingredients:

For the Salad:
• 1 cup cooked lentils, cooled
• 1 cup diced cucumber
• 1 cup diced tomatoes
• 1/2 cup diced bell pepper
• 1/2 cup diced red onion
• 2 tbsp chopped fresh parsley

For the Vinaigrette:
• 2 tbsp balsamic vinegar
• 1 tbsp olive oil
• 1 tsp Dijon mustard
• 1 tsp honey
• 1 garlic clove, minced
• Salt and pepper to taste

Instructions:

1. In a large bowl, combine the cooked lentils, cucumber, tomatoes, bell pepper, red onion, and parsley. Toss gently to mix.

2. In a small bowl, whisk together the balsamic vinegar, olive oil, Dijon mustard, honey, and garlic. Season with salt and pepper.

3. Pour the balsamic vinaigrette over the lentil salad and toss gently to coat.

4. Refrigerate the salad for at least 30 minutes to allow the flavors to meld.

5. Serve chilled or at room temperature.

This lentil salad is a great option for a fatty liver diet as lentils are a good source of plant•based protein, fiber, and complex carbohydrates. The mixed vegetables provide additional fiber, vitamins, and minerals, while the balsamic vinaigrette adds healthy fats and antioxidants. The overall dish is low in saturated fat and high in nutrients that can support liver health.

27. Turkey and black bean chili

Ingredients:

- 1 lb ground turkey
- 1 onion, diced
- 3 cloves garlic, minced
- 2 tbsp chili powder
- 1 tsp ground cumin
- 1 tsp dried oregano
- 1/2 tsp smoked paprika
- 1/4 tsp cayenne pepper (optional, for heat)
- 1 (15 oz) can black beans, rinsed and drained
- 1 (15 oz) can diced tomatoes
- 1 cup low•sodium chicken or vegetable broth
- Salt and pepper to taste
- Chopped fresh cilantro for garnish (optional)

Instructions:

1. In a large pot or Dutch oven, cook the ground turkey over medium•high heat, breaking it up with a wooden spoon, until browned and cooked through, about 5•7 minutes.

2. Add the diced onion and minced garlic to the pot. Cook for 2•3 minutes, until the onion is translucent.

3. Stir in the chili powder, cumin, oregano, smoked paprika, and cayenne (if using). Cook for 1 minute to toast the spices.

4. Add the black beans, diced tomatoes, and chicken/vegetable broth. Bring the mixture to a simmer and let it cook for 15•20 minutes, stirring occasionally, until the chili has thickened.

5. Season with salt and pepper to taste.

6. Serve the turkey and black bean chili hot, garnished with chopped fresh cilantro if desired.

This chili is a great option for a fatty liver diet as it is made with lean ground turkey, which is a low•fat protein source. The black beans provide fiber, protein, and complex carbohydrates. The spices and herbs add flavor without the need for excessive sodium or unhealthy fats.

28. Grilled chicken Caesar salad with a light dressing

Ingredients:

For the Salad:
- 4 boneless, skinless chicken breasts
- 1 romaine lettuce heart, chopped
- 1 cup cherry tomatoes, halved
- 1/4 cup shredded Parmesan cheese

For the Dressing:
- 2 tbsp plain Greek yogurt
- 1 tbsp lemon juice
- 1 tsp Dijon mustard
- 1 garlic clove, minced
- 1 tbsp olive oil
- 2 tbsp low•sodium chicken broth
- Salt and pepper to taste

Instructions:

1. Preheat grill or grill pan to medium•high heat.

2. Season the chicken breasts with salt and pepper. Grill for 5•7 minutes per side, until cooked through. Allow to cool slightly, then slice or shred the chicken.

3. In a large salad bowl, combine the chopped romaine lettuce, grilled chicken, cherry tomatoes, and Parmesan cheese.

4. In a small bowl, whisk together the Greek yogurt, lemon juice, Dijon mustard, garlic, olive oil, and chicken broth. Season with salt and pepper.

5. Drizzle the light Caesar dressing over the salad and toss gently to coat.

6. Serve the grilled chicken Caesar salad immediately.

This salad is a great option for a fatty liver diet as it is made with lean grilled chicken, nutrient•dense romaine lettuce, and a light, low•fat dressing. The Parmesan cheese provides a touch of flavor without adding excessive saturated fat. The overall dish is high in protein, fiber, and healthy fats, making it a balanced and liver•friendly meal.

29. Whole grain wrap with hummus, grilled chicken, and vegetables

Ingredients:

• 4 whole grain wraps or tortillas
• 1/2 cup hummus
• 1 lb boneless, skinless chicken breasts
• 1 cup sliced bell peppers
• 1 cup sliced cucumber
• 1 cup shredded carrots
• 1/4 cup crumbled feta cheese (optional)
• Salt and pepper to taste

Instructions:

1. Preheat grill or grill pan to medium•high heat.

2. Season the chicken breasts with salt and pepper. Grill for 5•7 minutes per side, until cooked through. Allow to cool slightly, then slice or shred the chicken.

3. Spread about 2 tablespoons of hummus onto each whole grain wrap or tortilla.

4. Top the hummus with the grilled chicken, sliced bell peppers, cucumber, and shredded carrots.

5. Sprinkle the crumbled feta cheese over the top, if using.

6. Fold the wrap or tortilla tightly around the filling and serve.

This wrap is a great option for a fatty liver diet as it combines lean protein from the grilled chicken, healthy fats from the hummus, and fiber•rich vegetables. The whole grain wrap provides complex carbohydrates and additional fiber. The overall dish is balanced and nutrient•dense, making it a liver•friendly meal.

You can customize the fillings to your liking, such as adding other crunchy vegetables or swapping the feta for a different cheese. This wrap is easy to prepare and can be enjoyed for a quick and healthy lunch or dinner.

30. Baked cod with a citrus glaze and steamed green beans

Ingredients:

For the Cod:
• 4 cod fillets (about 1 lb total)
• 2 tbsp fresh orange juice
• 1 tbsp fresh lemon juice
• 1 tbsp honey
• 1 tsp Dijon mustard
• 1 garlic clove, minced
• Salt and pepper to taste

For the Green Beans:
• 1 lb fresh green beans, trimmed
• 1 tbsp olive oil
• Salt and pepper to taste

Instructions:

1. Preheat oven to 400°F. Lightly grease a baking dish.

2. In a small bowl, whisk together the orange juice, lemon juice, honey, Dijon mustard, and garlic. Season with salt and pepper.

3. Place the cod fillets in the prepared baking dish and pour the citrus glaze over the top, making sure to coat the fish evenly.

4. Bake the cod for 15•18 minutes, or until it flakes easily with a fork.

5. While the cod is baking, steam the green beans until tender•crisp, about 5•7 minutes. Drain and toss with the olive oil, salt, and pepper.

6. Serve the baked cod immediately, drizzled with any remaining citrus glaze from the baking dish. Accompany with the steamed green beans.

This dish is an excellent choice for a fatty liver diet as cod is a lean, low•mercury fish that is high in protein and omega•3 fatty acids. The citrus glaze provides a burst of flavor without the need for excessive sodium or unhealthy fats. The steamed green beans are a nutrient•dense vegetable that is low in calories and high in fiber, vitamins, and minerals.

The overall meal is well•balanced, with a focus on lean protein, healthy fats, and fiber•rich vegetables • all of which can support liver health and function.

31. Zucchini noodles with marinara sauce and lean turkey meatballs

Ingredients:

For the Meatballs:
- 1 lb ground turkey
- 1/4 cup whole wheat breadcrumbs
- 1 egg, lightly beaten
- 2 tbsp grated Parmesan cheese
- 2 garlic cloves, minced
- 1 tsp dried oregano
- 1/2 tsp salt
- 1/4 tsp black pepper

For the Zucchini Noodles:
- 4 medium zucchinis, spiralized or julienned
- 1 tbsp olive oil
- 2 garlic cloves, minced
- 1 (24 oz) jar low•sodium marinara sauce

Instructions:

1. Preheat oven to 400°F. Line a baking sheet with parchment paper.

2. In a medium bowl, combine all the meatball ingredients and mix well. Roll the mixture into 1•inch meatballs and place them on the prepared baking sheet.

3. Bake the meatballs for 18•20 minutes, or until cooked through.

4. While the meatballs are baking, heat the olive oil in a large skillet over medium heat. Add the minced garlic and cook for 1 minute, until fragrant.

5. Add the spiralized or julienned zucchini noodles to the skillet and toss to coat with the garlic oil. Cook for 3•5 minutes, until the zucchini noodles are tender but still have a bite.

6. Pour the marinara sauce over the zucchini noodles and stir to combine. Simmer for 2•3 minutes to heat through. Serve the zucchini noodles with the baked turkey meatballs on top.

This dish is a great option for a fatty liver diet as it features lean ground turkey, which is a low•fat protein source. The zucchini noodles provide fiber, vitamins, and minerals, while the marinara sauce adds antioxidants from the tomatoes. The overall meal is low in saturated fat and high in nutrients that can support liver health.

32. Vegetable stir fry with tofu and brown rice

Ingredients:

For the Stir•Fry:
- 1 block (14 oz) extra•firm tofu, cubed
- 2 tbsp low•sodium soy sauce or tamari
- 1 tbsp sesame oil

For the Brown Rice:
- 1 cup uncooked brown rice
- 2 cups low•sodium vegetable or chicken broth

- 1 tbsp rice vinegar
- 1 tsp honey
- 1 tsp grated fresh ginger
- 2 cloves garlic, minced
- 1 red bell pepper, sliced
- 1 cup broccoli florets
- 1 cup sliced mushrooms
- 1 cup snow peas or snap peas
- 2 green onions, sliced

Instructions:

1. Cook the brown rice according to package instructions, using the broth instead of water.

2. In a small bowl, whisk together the soy sauce, sesame oil, rice vinegar, honey, ginger, and garlic. Set aside.

3. Heat a large wok or skillet over high heat. Add the cubed tofu and cook, stirring occasionally, until lightly browned on all sides, about 5•7 minutes. Transfer the tofu to a plate.

4. Add a splash of water or broth to the wok/skillet and stir•fry the bell pepper, broccoli, mushrooms, and snow/snap peas for 3•5 minutes, until tender•crisp.

5. Return the tofu to the wok/skillet and pour in the soy sauce mixture. Toss everything together and cook for 2•3 minutes, until the sauce has thickened slightly.

6. Remove from heat and stir in the sliced green onions. Serve the vegetable stir•fry over the cooked brown rice.

This stir•fry is a great option for a fatty liver diet as it features nutrient•dense vegetables, lean protein from the tofu, and whole grain brown rice. The soy sauce•based sauce provides flavor without excessive sodium. The overall dish is low in saturated fat and high in fiber, vitamins, and minerals that can support liver health.

33. Quinoa and black bean salad with avocado

Ingredients:

- 1 cup uncooked quinoa, rinsed
- 1 (15 oz) can black beans, rinsed and drained
- 1 cup diced cucumber
- 1 cup diced tomatoes
- 1/2 cup diced red onion
- 1 avocado, diced
- 2 tbsp chopped fresh cilantro
- 2 tbsp fresh lime juice
- 1 tbsp olive oil
- 1 tsp ground cumin
- Salt and pepper to taste

Instructions:

1. Cook the quinoa according to package instructions. Allow to cool completely.

2. In a large bowl, combine the cooked quinoa, black beans, cucumber, tomatoes, red onion, and avocado.

3. In a small bowl, whisk together the lime juice, olive oil, cumin, salt, and pepper.

4. Pour the dressing over the quinoa and bean salad and toss gently to coat.

5. Sprinkle the chopped fresh cilantro over the top.

6. Refrigerate the salad for at least 30 minutes to allow the flavors to meld.

7. Serve chilled or at room temperature.

This quinoa and black bean salad is an excellent choice for a fatty liver diet. Quinoa is a whole grain that is high in fiber, protein, and complex carbohydrates. Black beans provide additional fiber and plant•based protein. The avocado contributes healthy monounsaturated fats, while the vegetables and herbs add a variety of vitamins, minerals, and antioxidants.

The overall dish is well•balanced, nutrient•dense, and low in saturated fat, making it a great option to support liver health for women.

34. Baked chicken drumsticks with roasted root vegetables

Ingredients:

For the Chicken:
- 8 chicken drumsticks
- 1 tbsp olive oil
- 1 tsp paprika
- 1 tsp garlic powder
- Salt and pepper to taste

For the Vegetables:
- 2 cups cubed sweet potatoes
- 2 cups cubed carrots
- 1 cup cubed parsnips
- 1 red onion, cut into wedges
- 2 tbsp olive oil
- 1 tsp dried thyme
- Salt and pepper to taste

Instructions:

1. Preheat oven to 400°F. Line a large baking sheet with parchment paper.

2. In a large bowl, toss the chicken drumsticks with the olive oil, paprika, garlic powder, salt, and pepper until evenly coated.

3. Arrange the seasoned chicken drumsticks on one side of the prepared baking sheet.

4. In the same bowl, toss the cubed sweet potatoes, carrots, parsnips, and onion wedges with the olive oil, thyme, salt, and pepper.

5. Spread the seasoned root vegetables on the other side of the baking sheet, making sure they are in a single layer.

6. Bake for 35•40 minutes, flipping the chicken and stirring the vegetables halfway, until the chicken is cooked through and the vegetables are tender. Serve the baked chicken drumsticks with the roasted root vegetables.

This dish is a great option for a fatty liver diet as it features lean chicken drumsticks and a variety of nutrient•dense root vegetables. The chicken provides protein, while the vegetables offer fiber, complex carbohydrates, and a range of vitamins and minerals that can support liver health.

The baking method helps to keep the dish low in added fats, making it a healthier choice compared to fried or heavily sauced chicken dishes. This meal is well•balanced and can be easily customized with different types of root vegetables based on personal preferences.

35. Turkey and vegetable soup

Ingredients:

- 1 lb ground turkey
- 1 onion, diced
- 3 cloves garlic, minced
- 2 carrots, peeled and diced
- 2 celery stalks, diced
- 1 zucchini, diced
- 1 (15 oz) can diced tomatoes
- 4 cups low•sodium chicken or vegetable broth
- 1 tsp dried thyme
- 1 tsp dried oregano
- Salt and pepper to taste
- Chopped fresh parsley for garnish (optional)

Instructions:

1. In a large pot or Dutch oven, cook the ground turkey over medium•high heat, breaking it up with a wooden spoon, until browned and cooked through, about 5•7 minutes.

2. Add the diced onion and minced garlic to the pot. Cook for 2•3 minutes, until the onion is translucent.

3. Stir in the diced carrots, celery, and zucchini. Cook for 5 minutes, stirring occasionally.

4. Pour in the diced tomatoes and chicken/vegetable broth. Add the dried thyme and oregano. Season with salt and pepper to taste.

5. Bring the soup to a boil, then reduce the heat and let it simmer for 20•25 minutes, or until the vegetables are tender.

6. Ladle the turkey and vegetable soup into bowls and garnish with chopped fresh parsley, if desired.

This soup is an excellent choice for a fatty liver diet as it is made with lean ground turkey, which is a low•fat protein source. The variety of vegetables, including carrots, celery, zucchini, and tomatoes, provide fiber, vitamins, and antioxidants that can support liver health.

The broth•based soup is low in calories and fat, making it a nourishing and satisfying meal. You can adjust the seasoning to your taste preferences, and feel free to add any other vegetables you enjoy.

36. Greek yogurt with sliced fruit and a drizzle of honey

Ingredients:

• 1 cup plain Greek yogurt
• 1 cup sliced fresh fruit (such as berries, kiwi, mango, or pineapple)
• 1•2 tbsp honey

Instructions:

1. In a serving bowl or glass, layer the Greek yogurt and sliced fruit.

2. Drizzle the honey over the top of the yogurt and fruit.

3. Serve immediately or refrigerate until ready to enjoy.

This simple parfait is a great option for a fatty liver diet for a few reasons:

1. Greek yogurt is high in protein and low in fat, making it a great dairy choice. The protein helps keep you feeling full and satisfied.

2. Fresh fruit provides fiber, vitamins, and antioxidants that can support liver health. Choose a variety of colorful fruits for maximum nutritional benefits.

3. Honey is a natural sweetener that can be used in moderation to add a touch of sweetness without the need for refined sugars.

The combination of protein•rich yogurt, fiber•filled fruit, and a drizzle of honey creates a balanced and nourishing snack or light meal. This parfait is easy to prepare and can be customized with your favorite fruits.

Remember to enjoy this in moderation as part of an overall healthy, balanced diet that supports liver function for women with fatty liver disease.

37. Spinach and ricotta stuffed chicken breast

Ingredients:

• 4 boneless, skinless chicken breasts
• 1 cup part•skim ricotta cheese
• 1 cup fresh spinach, chopped
• 2 cloves garlic, minced
• 1/4 cup grated Parmesan cheese
• 1 tsp dried oregano
• Salt and pepper to taste

Instructions:

1. Preheat oven to 400°F. Lightly grease a baking dish.

2. In a medium bowl, mix together the ricotta cheese, chopped spinach, minced garlic, Parmesan cheese, and dried oregano. Season with salt and pepper.

3. Slice each chicken breast horizontally to create a pocket. Stuff each pocket with the ricotta•spinach mixture, dividing it evenly among the chicken breasts.

4. Place the stuffed chicken breasts in the prepared baking dish.

5. Bake for 25•30 minutes, or until the chicken is cooked through and the internal temperature reaches 165°F.

6. Serve the spinach and ricotta stuffed chicken breasts warm.

This dish is a great option for a fatty liver diet for a few reasons:

1. Chicken breast is a lean protein source that is low in saturated fat.
2. Spinach is a nutrient•dense green that is high in fiber, vitamins, and antioxidants.
3. Ricotta cheese provides protein and calcium without excessive fat.
4. The overall dish is baked, rather than fried, keeping it low in unhealthy fats.

The combination of lean protein, fiber•rich vegetables, and moderate amounts of dairy creates a well•balanced meal that can support liver health for women. You can serve this stuffed chicken with a side of roasted vegetables or a fresh salad for a complete and liver•friendly dinner.

38. Shrimp and vegetable stir fry with quinoa

Ingredients:

For the Stir•Fry:
• 1 lb raw shrimp, peeled and deveined
• 2 tbsp low•sodium soy sauce or tamari

For the Quinoa:
• 1 cup uncooked quinoa, rinsed
• 2 cups low•sodium vegetable or chicken broth

• 1 tbsp rice vinegar
• 1 tsp sesame oil
• 1 tsp honey
• 2 cloves garlic, minced
• 1 tbsp grated fresh ginger
• 1 red bell pepper, sliced
• 1 cup broccoli florets
• 1 cup sliced mushrooms
• 2 green onions, sliced

Instructions:

1. Cook the quinoa according to package instructions, using the broth instead of water.

2. In a small bowl, whisk together the soy sauce, rice vinegar, sesame oil, and honey. Set aside.

3. Heat a large wok or skillet over high heat. Add the shrimp and cook for 2•3 minutes, until they start to turn pink. Transfer the shrimp to a plate.

4. Add the minced garlic and grated ginger to the wok/skillet and cook for 1 minute, until fragrant.

5. Add the sliced bell pepper, broccoli, and mushrooms. Stir•fry for 3•5 minutes, until the vegetables are tender•crisp.

6. Return the cooked shrimp to the wok/skillet and pour in the soy sauce mixture. Toss everything together and cook for 2•3 minutes, until the sauce has thickened slightly.

7. Remove from heat and stir in the sliced green onions. Serve the shrimp and vegetable stir•fry over the cooked quinoa.

This dish is a great option for a fatty liver diet as it features lean protein from the shrimp, fiber•rich vegetables, and whole grain quinoa. The stir•fry is flavored with a light soy sauce•based sauce, providing flavor without excessive sodium.

The combination of protein, complex carbohydrates, and nutrient•dense vegetables makes this a well•balanced and liver•friendly meal. Quinoa is a great source of protein, fiber, and minerals that can support overall health.

39. Grilled portobello mushrooms with balsamic glaze

Ingredients:
- 4 large portobello mushroom caps, stems removed
- 2 tbsp olive oil
- 2 tbsp balsamic vinegar
- 1 tbsp honey
- 2 cloves garlic, minced
- 1 tsp dried thyme
- Salt and pepper to taste

Instructions:
1. Preheat grill or grill pan to medium·high heat.

2. In a small bowl, whisk together the olive oil, balsamic vinegar, honey, minced garlic, and dried thyme. Season with salt and pepper.

3. Brush the portobello mushroom caps on both sides with the balsamic glaze mixture, reserving any remaining glaze.

4. Grill the mushrooms for 4·5 minutes per side, or until they are tender and slightly charred. Transfer the grilled portobello mushrooms to a serving plate.

6. Drizzle any remaining balsamic glaze over the top of the mushrooms. Serve the grilled portobello mushrooms warm.

This dish is a great option for a fatty liver diet for a few reasons:

1. Portobello mushrooms are a low·calorie, low·fat, and high·fiber vegetable that can provide a satisfying "meaty" texture.

2. The balsamic vinegar and honey create a flavorful glaze without the need for excessive sodium or unhealthy fats.

3. Grilling the mushrooms helps to retain their nutrients and avoids the need for frying or sautéing in oil.

The overall dish is low in saturated fat and high in fiber, vitamins, and antioxidants that can support liver health for women. You can serve the grilled portobello mushrooms as a main dish or as a side to complement other lean protein sources.

40. Turkey and vegetable kebabs with a side of couscous

Ingredients:

For the Kebabs:
• 1 lb ground turkey
• 1 red bell pepper, cut into 1•inch pieces
• 1 zucchini, cut into 1•inch pieces
• 1 red onion, cut into 1•inch pieces
• 8 cherry tomatoes
• 2 tbsp olive oil
• 1 tsp dried oregano
• 1/2 tsp garlic powder
• Salt and pepper to taste

For the Couscous:
• 1 cup uncooked whole wheat couscous
• 1 cup low•sodium chicken or vegetable broth
• 2 tbsp chopped fresh parsley

Instructions:
1. Preheat grill or grill pan to medium•high heat.

2. In a large bowl, gently mix together the ground turkey, bell pepper, zucchini, onion, and cherry tomatoes. Drizzle with the olive oil and sprinkle with the oregano, garlic powder, salt, and pepper. Toss to coat.

3. Thread the turkey and vegetable mixture onto skewers, dividing evenly.

4. Grill the kebabs for 12•15 minutes, turning occasionally, until the turkey is cooked through and the vegetables are tender.

5. While the kebabs are grilling, prepare the couscous. Bring the broth to a boil in a small saucepan. Stir in the couscous, cover, and remove from heat. Let stand for 5 minutes, then fluff with a fork.

6. Serve the grilled turkey and vegetable kebabs over the cooked couscous, garnished with chopped fresh parsley.

This dish is a great option for a fatty liver diet as it features lean ground turkey, a variety of nutrient•dense vegetables, and whole grain couscous. The kebab format allows the flavors to meld together, while the grilling method keeps the dish low in added fats.

41. Baked salmon with a lemon dill sauce and steamed broccoli

Ingredients:

For the Salmon:
- 4 salmon fillets (about 1 lb total)
- 1 tbsp olive oil
- Salt and pepper to taste

For the Lemon•Dill Sauce:
- 1/4 cup plain Greek yogurt
- 2 tbsp fresh lemon juice
- 1 tbsp chopped fresh dill
- 1 garlic clove, minced
- Salt and pepper to taste

For the Broccoli:
- 1 lb broccoli florets
- 1 tbsp olive oil
- Salt and pepper to taste

Instructions:

1. Preheat oven to 400°F. Line a baking sheet with parchment paper.

2. Place the salmon fillets on the prepared baking sheet. Brush the top of the salmon with the olive oil and season with salt and pepper.

3. Bake the salmon for 12•15 minutes, or until it flakes easily with a fork.

4. While the salmon is baking, make the lemon•dill sauce. In a small bowl, whisk together the Greek yogurt, lemon juice, chopped dill, and minced garlic. Season with salt and pepper.

5. Steam the broccoli florets until tender•crisp, about 5•7 minutes. Toss the steamed broccoli with the olive oil, salt, and pepper.

6. Serve the baked salmon fillets with the lemon•dill sauce drizzled over the top. Accompany with the steamed broccoli.

The overall meal is well•balanced, with a focus on lean protein, healthy fats, and fiber•rich vegetables • all of which can support liver function and overall health for women.

42. Veggie packed egg muffins

Ingredients:

• 8 large eggs
• 1/2 cup diced bell pepper
• 1/2 cup diced spinach
• 1/4 cup diced onion
• 2 tbsp grated Parmesan cheese
• 1 tsp dried oregano
• Salt and pepper to taste

Instructions:

1. Preheat oven to 350°F. Grease a 12•cup muffin tin.

2. In a large bowl, whisk the eggs together. Stir in the diced bell pepper, spinach, onion, Parmesan cheese, oregano, salt, and pepper until well combined.

3. Divide the egg mixture evenly among the prepared muffin cups, filling each about 3/4 full.

4. Bake for 20•25 minutes, or until the egg muffins are set and lightly golden brown on top.

5. Allow the egg muffins to cool in the tin for 5 minutes before removing them.

6. Serve the veggie•packed egg muffins warm or at room temperature.

These egg muffins are a great option for a fatty liver diet for a few reasons:

1. Eggs are a lean protein source that are low in saturated fat.

2. The vegetables, including bell pepper, spinach, and onion, provide fiber, vitamins, and antioxidants that can support liver health.

3. The small portion size and baked preparation method keep the dish low in added fats.

You can customize the veggie fillings based on your preferences or what you have on hand. The egg muffins can be made in advance and reheated for a quick and nutritious breakfast or snack.

Pair these egg muffins with a side of fresh fruit or a small serving of whole grain toast for a complete and liver•friendly meal.

43. Turkey lettuce wraps with a side of quinoa

Ingredients:

For the Turkey Wraps:
• 1 lb ground turkey
• 1 tbsp olive oil
• 1 onion, diced
• 2 cloves garlic, minced
• 1 tbsp low•sodium soy sauce or tamari
• 1 tsp ground cumin
• 1/2 tsp chili powder
• Salt and pepper to taste
• 12 large lettuce leaves (such as romaine or bibb)

For the Quinoa:
• 1 cup uncooked quinoa, rinsed
• 2 cups low•sodium chicken or vegetable broth

Instructions:

1. Cook the quinoa according to package instructions, using the broth instead of water.

2. In a large skillet, heat the olive oil over medium•high heat. Add the ground turkey and cook, breaking it up with a wooden spoon, until browned and cooked through, about 5•7 minutes.

3. Add the diced onion and minced garlic to the skillet. Cook for 2•3 minutes, until the onion is translucent.

4. Stir in the soy sauce, cumin, chili powder, salt, and pepper. Cook for 1•2 minutes to allow the flavors to blend.

5. To serve, place a couple of tablespoons of the turkey mixture into the center of a lettuce leaf. Fold the lettuce around the filling to create a wrap. Serve the turkey lettuce wraps with the cooked quinoa on the side.

This dish is a great option for a fatty liver diet for the following reasons:

1. Ground turkey is a lean protein source that is low in saturated fat.
2. Lettuce leaves provide a low•calorie, fiber•rich wrap for the turkey filling.
3. Quinoa is a whole grain that is high in protein, fiber, and complex carbohydrates.
4. The overall dish is low in added fats and sodium, making it a healthier choice.

44. Lentil and vegetable curry with brown rice

Ingredients:

For the Curry:
- 1 cup dry brown lentils, rinsed
- 2 cups low•sodium vegetable broth
- 1 tbsp olive oil
- 1 onion, diced
- 3 cloves garlic, minced
- 1 tbsp grated fresh ginger
- 2 tsp curry powder
- 1 tsp ground cumin
- 1/2 tsp ground turmeric
- 1 (14 oz) can diced tomatoes
- 1 cup diced cauliflower
- 1 cup diced sweet potato
- 1 cup frozen peas
- Salt and pepper to taste

For the Brown Rice:
- 1 cup uncooked brown rice
- 2 cups low•sodium vegetable or chicken broth

Instructions:

1. Cook the brown rice according to package instructions, using the broth instead of water.

2. In a large pot, combine the rinsed lentils and vegetable broth. Bring to a boil, then reduce heat and simmer for 15•20 minutes, until the lentils are tender.

3. In a separate skillet, heat the olive oil over medium heat. Add the diced onion, minced garlic, and grated ginger. Cook for 2•3 minutes, until fragrant.

4. Stir in the curry powder, cumin, and turmeric. Cook for 1 minute to toast the spices.

5. Add the diced tomatoes, cauliflower, sweet potato, and frozen peas to the skillet. Simmer for 10•15 minutes, until the vegetables are tender.

6. Drain the cooked lentils and add them to the vegetable curry. Season with salt and pepper to taste. Serve the lentil and vegetable curry over the cooked brown rice.

The overall meal is well•balanced, low in saturated fat, and high in fiber, vitamins, and minerals that can support liver health for women.

45. Grilled chicken with roasted vegetables and a side of quinoa

Ingredients:

For the Chicken:
• 4 boneless, skinless chicken breasts
• 1 tbsp olive oil
• 1 tsp dried oregano
• Salt and pepper to taste

For the Quinoa:
• 1 cup uncooked quinoa, rinsed
• 2 cups low•sodium chicken or vegetable broth

For the Roasted Vegetables:
• 2 cups cubed sweet potatoes
• 2 cups broccoli florets
• 1 red bell pepper, diced
• 1 red onion, diced
• 2 tbsp olive oil
• 1 tsp dried thyme
• Salt and pepper to taste

Instructions:

1. Preheat grill or grill pan to medium•high heat.

2. Prepare the quinoa according to package instructions, using the broth instead of water.

3. In a large bowl, toss the cubed sweet potatoes, broccoli florets, bell pepper, and onion with the olive oil, thyme, salt, and pepper.

4. Spread the seasoned vegetables in a single layer on a baking sheet. Roast at 400°F for 20•25 minutes, stirring halfway, until the vegetables are tender and lightly browned.

5. While the vegetables are roasting, brush the chicken breasts with the olive oil and season with the oregano, salt, and pepper.

6. Grill the chicken for 5•7 minutes per side, or until cooked through and no longer pink in the center. Serve the grilled chicken alongside the roasted vegetables and cooked quinoa.

The combination of lean protein, fiber•rich vegetables, and complex carbohydrates creates a well•balanced and nutrient•dense meal that can support liver health for women. The grilling and roasting methods also help to keep the dish low in added fats.

46. Tofu and vegetable stir fry with brown rice

Ingredients:

For the Stir•Fry:
- 1 block (14 oz) extra•firm tofu, cubed
- 2 tbsp low•sodium soy sauce or tamari
- 1 tbsp sesame oil

For the Brown Rice:
- 1 cup uncooked brown rice
- 2 cups low•sodium vegetable or chicken broth

- 1 tbsp rice vinegar
- 1 tsp honey
- 2 cloves garlic, minced
- 1 tbsp grated fresh ginger
- 1 red bell pepper, sliced
- 1 cup broccoli florets
- 1 cup sliced mushrooms
- 1 cup snow peas or snap peas
- 2 green onions, sliced

Instructions:

1. Cook the brown rice according to package instructions, using the broth instead of water.

2. In a small bowl, whisk together the soy sauce, sesame oil, rice vinegar, and honey. Set aside.

3. Heat a large wok or skillet over high heat. Add the cubed tofu and cook, stirring occasionally, until lightly browned on all sides, about 5•7 minutes. Transfer the tofu to a plate.

4. Add the minced garlic and grated ginger to the wok/skillet. Cook for 1 minute, until fragrant.

5. Add the sliced bell pepper, broccoli, mushrooms, and snow/snap peas. Stir•fry for 3•5 minutes, until the vegetables are tender•crisp.

6. Return the tofu to the wok/skillet and pour in the soy sauce mixture. Toss everything together and cook for 2•3 minutes, until the sauce has thickened slightly.

7. Remove from heat and stir in the sliced green onions. Serve the tofu and vegetable stir•fry over the cooked brown rice.

The overall meal is well•balanced, low in saturated fat, and high in fiber, vitamins, and minerals that can support liver health for women. You can adjust the vegetable selection based on your preferences.

47. Stuffed bell peppers with ground turkey and quinoa

Ingredients:

- 4 large bell peppers, halved and seeded
- 1 lb ground turkey
- 1 cup cooked quinoa
- 1 onion, diced
- 2 cloves garlic, minced
- 1 (14.5 oz) can diced tomatoes
- 1 tsp dried oregano
- 1/2 tsp ground cumin
- Salt and pepper to taste
- 1/4 cup shredded mozzarella cheese (optional)

Instructions:

1. Preheat oven to 375°F. Lightly grease a baking dish.

2. Arrange the bell pepper halves in the prepared baking dish.

3. In a large skillet, cook the ground turkey over medium•high heat, breaking it up with a wooden spoon, until browned and cooked through, about 5•7 minutes.

4. Add the diced onion and minced garlic to the skillet. Cook for 2•3 minutes, until the onion is translucent.

5. Stir in the cooked quinoa, diced tomatoes, oregano, cumin, salt, and pepper. Cook for 5 minutes, allowing the flavors to blend.

6. Spoon the turkey and quinoa mixture into the bell pepper halves, dividing it evenly.

7. If desired, sprinkle the tops of the stuffed peppers with the shredded mozzarella cheese.

8. Bake for 25•30 minutes, or until the peppers are tender and the filling is hot.

9. Serve the stuffed bell peppers warm.

The combination of lean protein, complex carbohydrates, and fiber•rich vegetables creates a well•balanced and liver•friendly meal. You can adjust the spices or add other vegetables to the filling based on your preferences.

48. Baked cod with roasted cherry tomatoes and green beans

Ingredients:

For the Cod:
- 4 cod fillets (about 1 lb total)
- 1 tbsp olive oil
- 1 tsp lemon zest
- 1 tbsp fresh lemon juice
- 1 tsp dried parsley
- Salt and pepper to taste

For the Roasted Vegetables:
- 1 pint cherry tomatoes, halved
- 1 lb fresh green beans, trimmed
- 2 tbsp olive oil
- 1 tsp dried thyme
- Salt and pepper to taste

Instructions:

1. Preheat oven to 400°F. Line a baking sheet with parchment paper.

2. In a small bowl, mix together the olive oil, lemon zest, lemon juice, and dried parsley. Season the cod fillets with salt and pepper, then brush the top of each fillet with the lemon•herb mixture.

3. Place the cod fillets on one side of the prepared baking sheet.

4. In a separate bowl, toss the halved cherry tomatoes and trimmed green beans with the olive oil, dried thyme, salt, and pepper.

5. Spread the seasoned vegetables on the other side of the baking sheet, making sure they are in a single layer.

6. Bake for 18•22 minutes, or until the cod is cooked through and flakes easily with a fork, and the vegetables are tender.

7. Serve the baked cod immediately, with the roasted cherry tomatoes and green beans on the side.

The combination of the baked cod, roasted vegetables, and simple lemon•herb seasoning creates a well•balanced and liver•friendly meal. You can adjust the cooking time based on the thickness of your cod fillets.

49. Lentil and kale salad
with a lemon tahini dressing

Ingredients:
For the Salad:
• 1 cup cooked lentils, cooled
• 4 cups chopped kale
• 1 cup diced cucumber
• 1/2 cup diced red onion
• 1/4 cup chopped fresh parsley

For the Dressing:
• 2 tbsp tahini
• 2 tbsp fresh lemon juice
• 1 tbsp olive oil
• 1 tsp honey
• 1 garlic clove, minced
• 2•3 tbsp water, as needed
• Salt and pepper to taste

Instructions:
1. In a large bowl, combine the cooked lentils, chopped kale, diced cucumber, red onion, and chopped parsley. Toss to mix.

2. In a small bowl, whisk together the tahini, lemon juice, olive oil, honey, and minced garlic. Add water, 1 tbsp at a time, until the dressing reaches your desired consistency. Season with salt and pepper.

3. Pour the lemon•tahini dressing over the lentil and kale salad. Toss gently to coat.

4. Refrigerate the salad for at least 30 minutes to allow the flavors to meld.

5. Serve the lentil and kale salad chilled or at room temperature.

You can customize the salad by adding other vegetables or herbs that you enjoy. The lentil and kale combination, paired with the flavorful dressing, makes for a nourishing and liver•friendly meal.

50. Turkey and vegetable stir fry with soba noodles

Ingredients:

- 8 oz soba noodles
- 1 lb ground turkey
- 2 tbsp low•sodium soy sauce or tamari
- 1 tbsp rice vinegar
- 1 tsp sesame oil
- 1 tsp honey
- 2 cloves garlic, minced
- 1 tbsp grated fresh ginger
- 1 red bell pepper, sliced
- 1 cup broccoli florets
- 1 cup sliced mushrooms
- 2 green onions, sliced

Instructions:

1. Cook the soba noodles according to package instructions. Drain and rinse with cold water.

2. In a small bowl, whisk together the soy sauce, rice vinegar, sesame oil, and honey. Set aside.

3. Heat a large wok or skillet over high heat. Add the ground turkey and cook, breaking it up with a wooden spoon, until browned and cooked through, about 5•7 minutes.

4. Add the minced garlic and grated ginger to the wok/skillet. Cook for 1 minute, until fragrant.

5. Stir in the sliced bell pepper, broccoli florets, and mushrooms. Stir•fry for 3•5 minutes, until the vegetables are tender•crisp.

6. Add the cooked soba noodles and the soy sauce mixture to the wok/skillet. Toss everything together and cook for 2•3 minutes, until the noodles are heated through and the sauce has thickened slightly.

7. Remove from heat and stir in the sliced green onions. Serve the turkey and vegetable stir•fry with soba noodles immediately.

The combination of lean protein, whole grains, and fiber•rich vegetables creates a well•balanced and liver•friendly meal. You can adjust the vegetable selection based on your preferences.

51. Grilled shrimp skewers with a mango salsa

Ingredients:

• 1 lb large shrimp, peeled and deveined
• 1 mango, diced
• 1/2 red onion, finely chopped
• 1 jalapeño, seeded and finely chopped
• 1/4 cup chopped fresh cilantro
• 2 tbsp lime juice
• 1 tbsp olive oil
• Salt and pepper to taste

Instructions:

1. In a medium bowl, combine the diced mango, red onion, jalapeño, cilantro, lime juice, and a pinch of salt and pepper. Stir to mix well and set aside.

2. Thread the shrimp onto skewers, leaving a little space between each one.

3. Brush the shrimp lightly with olive oil and season with salt and pepper.

4. Grill the shrimp skewers over medium•high heat for 2•3 minutes per side, until the shrimp are opaque and cooked through.

5. Serve the grilled shrimp skewers immediately, topped with the fresh mango salsa.

This recipe is supportive for a fatty liver diet for women for a few reasons:

• Shrimp is a lean protein that is low in saturated fat, which is important for fatty liver disease.

• Mango is a fruit high in fiber, vitamins, and antioxidants that can help support liver health.

• The olive oil provides healthy unsaturated fats.

• The dish is light and fresh, without heavy sauces or fried elements.

The combination of lean protein, fresh produce, and healthy fats makes this a great option for a fatty liver•friendly meal. Enjoy!

52. Baked chicken breast
with a Mediterranean quinoa salad

Ingredients:

Chicken:
• 4 boneless, skinless chicken breasts
• 1 tbsp olive oil
• 1 tsp dried oregano
• Salt and pepper to taste

Quinoa Salad:
• 1 cup uncooked quinoa, rinsed
• 1 cup cherry tomatoes, halved
• 1/2 cup diced cucumber
• 1/4 cup crumbled feta cheese
• 1/4 cup chopped kalamata olives
• 2 tbsp chopped fresh parsley
• 2 tbsp lemon juice
• 1 tbsp olive oil
• 1 garlic clove, minced
• Salt and pepper to taste

Instructions:

1. Preheat the oven to 400°F. Season the chicken breasts with the oregano, salt, and pepper. Place in a baking dish and drizzle with 1 tbsp of olive oil.

2. Bake the chicken for 25•30 minutes, until cooked through and no longer pink in the center.

3. While the chicken is baking, cook the quinoa according to package instructions. Allow to cool slightly.

4. In a large bowl, combine the cooked quinoa, cherry tomatoes, cucumber, feta, olives, and parsley.

5. In a small bowl, whisk together the lemon juice, 1 tbsp olive oil, and minced garlic. Season with salt and pepper. Pour the dressing over the quinoa salad and toss to coat. Serve the baked chicken breasts warm, topped with the Mediterranean quinoa salad.

The combination of lean protein, whole grains, and nutrient•dense vegetables makes this a great option for a fatty liver•friendly meal. Enjoy!

53. Eggplant and chickpea curry with brown rice

Ingredients:

Curry:
• 1 medium eggplant, cubed
• 1 (15 oz) can chickpeas, drained and rinsed
• 1 onion, diced
• 3 cloves garlic, minced
• 1 tbsp grated fresh ginger
• 2 tsp curry powder
• 1 tsp ground cumin
• 1 tsp ground coriander
• 1 (14 oz) can diced tomatoes
• 1 cup low•sodium vegetable broth
• 1 cup full•fat coconut milk
• Salt and pepper to taste
• Chopped cilantro for garnish

Brown Rice:
• 1 cup uncooked brown rice
• 2 cups low•sodium vegetable broth

Instructions:

1. Cook the brown rice: In a medium saucepan, bring the 2 cups of vegetable broth to a boil. Add the brown rice, cover, reduce heat to low and simmer for 25•30 minutes until rice is tender. Fluff with a fork.

2. Make the curry: In a large skillet or Dutch oven, sauté the onion in a splash of vegetable broth over medium heat for 5 minutes until translucent.

3. Add the garlic and ginger and cook for 1 minute until fragrant.

4. Stir in the curry powder, cumin, and coriander and cook for 1 minute.

5. Add the eggplant, chickpeas, diced tomatoes, vegetable broth, and coconut milk. Bring to a simmer and cook for 15•20 minutes, until the eggplant is very soft.

6. Season the curry with salt and pepper to taste. Serve the eggplant and chickpea curry over the cooked brown rice. Garnish with chopped cilantro.

The combination of fiber•rich vegetables, lean plant•based protein, and whole grains makes this a great option for a fatty liver•friendly meal. Enjoy!

54. Spinach and feta stuffed turkey burgers

Ingredients:

Burgers:
• 1 lb ground turkey
• 1 cup fresh spinach, chopped
• 1/2 cup crumbled feta cheese
• 1 egg, lightly beaten
• 2 tbsp whole wheat breadcrumbs
• 1 tsp dried oregano
• 1/2 tsp garlic powder
• Salt and pepper to taste

For Serving:
• Whole wheat buns
• Lettuce, tomato, onion (optional toppings)

Instructions:

1. In a large bowl, combine the ground turkey, chopped spinach, feta cheese, egg, breadcrumbs, oregano, garlic powder, salt, and pepper. Mix gently until just combined, being careful not to overmix.

2. Divide the turkey mixture into 4 equal portions and shape each into a patty, making a small indent in the center of each one.

3. Preheat a grill or grill pan over medium•high heat. Cook the burgers for 4•5 minutes per side, until cooked through and no longer pink in the center.

4. Serve the spinach and feta stuffed turkey burgers on whole wheat buns, topped with lettuce, tomato, onion, or any other desired toppings.

This recipe is supportive for a fatty liver diet for women for a few reasons:

• Ground turkey is a lean protein that is low in saturated fat, which is important for fatty liver disease.
• Spinach is a nutrient•dense green that is high in fiber, vitamins, and antioxidants to support liver health.
• Feta cheese provides a source of healthy fat without being too high in saturated fat.
• Whole wheat buns are a whole grain option that is higher in fiber compared to refined white buns.

55. Baked tilapia with a pineapple salsa and steamed asparagus

Ingredients:

Tilapia:
- 4 tilapia fillets
- 1 tbsp olive oil
- 1 tsp paprika
- Salt and pepper to taste

Asparagus:
- 1 lb asparagus spears, trimmed
- 1 tbsp water

Pineapple Salsa:
- 1 cup diced fresh pineapple
- 1/2 red onion, diced
- 1 jalapeño, seeded and diced
- 2 tbsp chopped fresh cilantro
- 1 tbsp lime juice
- Salt and pepper to taste

Instructions:

1. Preheat the oven to 400°F. Place the tilapia fillets in a baking dish and drizzle with the olive oil. Sprinkle with paprika, salt, and pepper.

2. Bake the tilapia for 15•18 minutes, until it flakes easily with a fork.

3. While the tilapia is baking, make the pineapple salsa. In a medium bowl, combine the diced pineapple, red onion, jalapeño, cilantro, and lime juice. Season with salt and pepper to taste.

4. Steam the asparagus: Place the asparagus spears in a steamer basket set over a pot of simmering water. Cover and steam for 5•7 minutes, until tender•crisp.

5. Serve the baked tilapia topped with the pineapple salsa, alongside the steamed asparagus.

This recipe is supportive for a fatty liver diet for women for a few reasons:

- Tilapia is a lean, mild•flavored fish that is low in mercury and high in protein.
- Pineapple is a fruit that is high in fiber, vitamins, and antioxidants to support liver health.
- Asparagus is a vegetable that is high in fiber, folate, and antioxidants.
- The dish is baked and steamed, avoiding any fried or high•fat cooking methods.

The combination of lean protein, fresh produce, and healthy cooking methods makes this a great option for a fatty liver•friendly meal. Enjoy!

56. Lentil and vegetable soup

Ingredients:

• 1 cup dry brown or green lentils, rinsed
• 1 tbsp olive oil
• 1 onion, diced
• 3 carrots, peeled and diced
• 3 celery stalks, diced
• 3 garlic cloves, minced
• 1 tsp ground cumin
• 1 tsp dried oregano
• 1/2 tsp smoked paprika
• 4 cups low•sodium vegetable broth
• 1 (14 oz) can diced tomatoes
• 2 cups chopped kale or spinach
• Salt and pepper to taste
• Chopped parsley for garnish (optional)

Instructions:

1. In a large pot or Dutch oven, heat the olive oil over medium heat. Add the onion, carrots, and celery. Sauté for 5•7 minutes until the vegetables start to soften.

2. Add the garlic, cumin, oregano, and smoked paprika. Cook for 1 minute until fragrant.

3. Pour in the vegetable broth and diced tomatoes. Bring the soup to a boil.

4. Add the rinsed lentils and reduce the heat to medium•low. Simmer for 20•25 minutes, until the lentils are tender.

5. Stir in the chopped kale or spinach and cook for 2•3 minutes until the greens are wilted.

6. Season the soup with salt and pepper to taste.

7. Ladle the lentil and vegetable soup into bowls and garnish with chopped parsley if desired.

The combination of fiber•rich lentils, nutrient•dense vegetables, and a simple broth•based preparation makes this lentil and vegetable soup an excellent option for a fatty liver•friendly diet. Enjoy!

57. Greek yogurt with sliced banana and almonds

Ingredients:
• 1 cup plain Greek yogurt
• 1 medium banana, sliced
• 2 tbsp sliced or slivered almonds

Instructions:
1. Spoon the Greek yogurt into a bowl or serving dish.

2. Top the yogurt with the sliced banana.

3. Sprinkle the sliced almonds over the top.

That's it! This simple dish provides a nutritious combination of ingredients that can be beneficial for a fatty liver diet for women.

Here's why this recipe is supportive:

• Greek yogurt is an excellent source of protein, which is important for maintaining muscle mass and supporting overall health. It's also lower in fat compared to regular yogurt.

• Bananas are a good source of fiber, vitamins, and potassium. The fiber can help support digestive and liver health.

• Almonds are a healthy source of unsaturated fats, fiber, and antioxidants. The healthy fats and fiber can help promote feelings of fullness.

The combination of protein•rich Greek yogurt, fiber•filled banana, and heart•healthy almonds makes this a nutrient•dense snack or light meal that can be beneficial for women managing fatty liver disease. It's easy to prepare and provides a satisfying texture and flavor profile.

58. Quinoa and black bean stuffed bell peppers

Ingredients:

- 4 medium bell peppers, halved lengthwise and seeds removed
- 1 cup cooked quinoa
- 1 (15 oz) can black beans, rinsed and drained
- 1 cup diced tomatoes
- 1/2 cup crumbled feta cheese
- 2 tbsp chopped fresh cilantro
- 1 tsp ground cumin
- 1/2 tsp garlic powder
- Salt and pepper to taste

Instructions:

1. Preheat the oven to 375°F. Place the bell pepper halves in a baking dish and set aside.

2. In a medium bowl, combine the cooked quinoa, black beans, diced tomatoes, feta cheese, cilantro, cumin, garlic powder, salt, and pepper. Stir to mix well.

3. Spoon the quinoa and black bean mixture evenly into the bell pepper halves.

4. Cover the baking dish with foil and bake for 25•30 minutes, until the peppers are tender.

5. Remove the foil and bake for an additional 5 minutes to lightly brown the tops. Serve the stuffed bell peppers warm.

This recipe is supportive for a fatty liver diet for women for a few reasons:

- Quinoa is a whole grain that is high in fiber, protein, and nutrients.

- Black beans are a great source of plant•based protein and fiber.

- Bell peppers are packed with vitamins, minerals, and antioxidants.

- Feta cheese provides a source of healthy fat without being too high in saturated fat.

- The dish is baked, not fried, keeping it light and healthy.

The combination of whole grains, lean protein, vegetables, and healthy fats makes this a nutritious and filling meal that can be beneficial for women managing fatty liver disease.

59. Grilled chicken and vegetable kabobs with quinoa

Ingredients:
Kabobs:
• 1 lb boneless, skinless chicken breasts, cut into 1•inch cubes
• 1 zucchini, cut into 1•inch pieces
• 1 red bell pepper, cut into 1•inch pieces
• 1 yellow onion, cut into 1•inch pieces
• 8 oz mushrooms, halved
• 2 tbsp olive oil
• 1 tsp dried oregano
• 1/2 tsp garlic powder
• Salt and pepper to taste

Quinoa:
• 1 cup uncooked quinoa, rinsed
• 2 cups low•sodium vegetable or chicken broth

Instructions:
1. Preheat grill to medium•high heat.

2. In a large bowl, toss the chicken and vegetables with the olive oil, oregano, garlic powder, salt, and pepper until evenly coated.

3. Thread the chicken and vegetables onto skewers, alternating the ingredients.

4. Grill the kabobs for 12•15 minutes, turning occasionally, until the chicken is cooked through and the vegetables are tender.

5. While the kabobs are grilling, cook the quinoa. In a medium saucepan, bring the broth to a boil. Add the quinoa, cover, reduce heat to low and simmer for 15•20 minutes until the quinoa is tender and the liquid is absorbed. Serve the grilled chicken and vegetable kabobs over the cooked quinoa.

This recipe is supportive for a fatty liver diet for women for a few reasons:

• Chicken breast is a lean protein that is low in saturated fat.
• Vegetables like zucchini, bell pepper, onion, and mushrooms are high in fiber, vitamins, and antioxidants.
• Quinoa is a whole grain that is high in fiber, protein, and nutrients.
• The dish is grilled, which is a healthy cooking method that doesn't require added oils or fats.

60. Tofu and broccoli stir fry with brown rice

Ingredients:

Stir•Fry:
• 1 block extra•firm tofu, pressed and cubed
• 3 cups broccoli florets
• 1 red bell pepper, sliced
• 1 cup sliced mushrooms
• 2 cloves garlic, minced
• 1 tbsp grated fresh ginger
• 2 tbsp low•sodium soy sauce or tamari
• 1 tbsp rice vinegar
• 1 tsp sesame oil
• 1 tsp cornstarch
• Salt and pepper to taste

Brown Rice:
• 1 cup uncooked brown rice
• 2 cups low•sodium vegetable or chicken broth

Instructions:

1. Cook the brown rice: In a medium saucepan, bring the broth to a boil. Add the brown rice, cover, reduce heat to low and simmer for 25•30 minutes until rice is tender.

2. Make the stir•fry: In a large skillet or wok, heat 1 tsp of sesame oil over medium•high heat. Add the cubed tofu and cook for 3•4 minutes per side until lightly browned. Remove tofu from the pan and set aside.

3. In the same pan, add another 1 tsp of sesame oil. Add the broccoli, bell pepper, and mushrooms. Stir•fry for 5•7 minutes until vegetables are tender•crisp.

4. Add the garlic and ginger and cook for 1 minute until fragrant.

5. In a small bowl, whisk together the soy sauce, rice vinegar, and cornstarch. Pour the sauce into the pan and let it simmer for 2•3 minutes until thickened slightly.

6. Return the cooked tofu to the pan and toss everything together until well coated. Serve the tofu and broccoli stir•fry over the cooked brown rice.

The combination of plant•based protein, fiber•rich vegetables, and whole grains makes this tofu and broccoli stir•fry a great option for a fatty liver•friendly meal. Enjoy!

61. Turkey and vegetable lettuce wraps with a side of quinoa

Ingredients:

Lettuce Wraps:
• 1 lb ground turkey
• 1 cup diced mushrooms
• 1 cup diced bell pepper
• 1 cup shredded carrots
• 2 cloves garlic, minced
• 1 tbsp low•sodium soy sauce or tamari
• 1 tsp sesame oil
• 1/2 tsp ground ginger
• Salt and pepper to taste
• Bibb or romaine lettuce leaves for wrapping

Quinoa:
• 1 cup uncooked quinoa, rinsed
• 2 cups low•sodium vegetable or chicken broth

Instructions:

1. Cook the quinoa: In a medium saucepan, bring the broth to a boil. Add the quinoa, cover, reduce heat to low and simmer for 15•20 minutes until quinoa is tender and liquid is absorbed.

2. Make the lettuce wraps: In a large skillet over medium•high heat, cook the ground turkey, breaking it up with a wooden spoon, until no longer pink, about 5•7 minutes.

3. Add the mushrooms, bell pepper, carrots, garlic, soy sauce, sesame oil, and ginger. Stir•fry for 5•7 minutes until the vegetables are tender.

4. Season the turkey and vegetable mixture with salt and pepper to taste.

5. To serve, spoon the turkey and vegetable mixture into the lettuce leaves. Serve with the cooked quinoa on the side.

The combination of lean protein, fiber•rich vegetables, and nutrient•dense whole grains makes this a well•balanced and liver•friendly meal. Enjoy!

62. Lentil and spinach salad with a balsamic vinaigrette

Ingredients:

Salad:
- 1 cup cooked lentils, cooled
- 4 cups fresh spinach, chopped
- 1/2 cup diced cucumber
- 1/4 cup diced red onion
- 2 tbsp crumbled feta cheese

Vinaigrette:
- 2 tbsp balsamic vinegar
- 1 tbsp olive oil
- 1 tsp Dijon mustard
- 1 tsp honey
- 1 garlic clove, minced
- Salt and pepper to taste

Instructions:

1. In a large bowl, combine the cooked lentils, spinach, cucumber, red onion, and feta cheese.

2. In a small bowl, whisk together the balsamic vinegar, olive oil, Dijon mustard, honey, and minced garlic. Season with salt and pepper.

3. Drizzle the balsamic vinaigrette over the lentil and spinach salad and toss gently to coat. Serve the lentil and spinach salad immediately.

This recipe is supportive for a fatty liver diet for women for a few reasons:

- Lentils are a great source of plant•based protein and fiber, which can help support liver health.
- Spinach is a nutrient•dense green that is high in vitamins, minerals, and antioxidants.
- The balsamic vinaigrette provides a flavorful dressing without relying on high•fat ingredients.
- Feta cheese adds a small amount of healthy fat without being too high in saturated fat.
- The dish is light, fresh, and vegetable•forward, making it a great option for a fatty liver•friendly meal.

The combination of fiber•rich lentils, leafy greens, and a simple vinaigrette dressing makes this lentil and spinach salad a nutritious and delicious choice for women managing fatty liver disease. Enjoy!

63. Baked cod with roasted vegetables and quinoa

Ingredients:

Roasted Vegetables:
• 1 lb Brussels sprouts, trimmed and halved
• 1 medium zucchini, diced
• 1 red bell pepper, diced
• 1 red onion, diced
• 2 tbsp olive oil
• Salt and pepper to taste

Cod:
• 4 (6 oz) cod fillets
• 1 tbsp olive oil
• 1 tsp paprika
• 1/2 tsp garlic powder
• Salt and pepper to taste

Quinoa:
• 1 cup uncooked quinoa, rinsed
• 2 cups low•sodium vegetable or chicken broth

Instructions:
1. Preheat the oven to 400°F.

2. Prepare the roasted vegetables: In a large baking dish, toss the Brussels sprouts, zucchini, bell pepper, and onion with the 2 tbsp of olive oil. Season with salt and pepper. Roast for 20•25 minutes, stirring halfway, until vegetables are tender and lightly browned.

3. While the vegetables are roasting, cook the quinoa. In a medium saucepan, bring the broth to a boil. Add the quinoa, cover, reduce heat to low and simmer for 15•20 minutes until quinoa is tender and liquid is absorbed.

4. Season the cod fillets with the paprika, garlic powder, salt, and pepper. Place the cod on a baking sheet and bake for 12•15 minutes, until the fish flakes easily with a fork.

5. To serve, place a portion of the roasted vegetables and a cod fillet on a bed of the cooked quinoa.

The combination of lean protein, fiber•rich vegetables, and nutrient•dense whole grains makes this a well•balanced and liver•friendly meal. Enjoy!

64. Turkey and vegetable stir fry with whole wheat noodles

Ingredients:

Stir•Fry:
- 1 lb ground turkey
- 2 cups broccoli florets
- 1 red bell pepper, sliced
- 1 cup sliced mushrooms
- 1 cup shredded carrots
- 2 cloves garlic, minced
- 1 tbsp grated fresh ginger
- 2 tbsp low•sodium soy sauce or tamari
- 1 tbsp rice vinegar
- 1 tsp sesame oil
- Salt and pepper to taste

Noodles:
- 8 oz whole wheat spaghetti or linguine
- 2 cups low•sodium vegetable or chicken broth

Instructions:

1. Bring a large pot of water to a boil. Cook the whole wheat noodles according to package instructions until al dente. Drain and set aside.

2. In a large skillet or wok, cook the ground turkey over medium•high heat, breaking it up with a wooden spoon, until no longer pink, about 5•7 minutes.

3. Add the broccoli, bell pepper, mushrooms, and carrots to the skillet. Stir•fry for 5•7 minutes until the vegetables are tender•crisp.

4. Stir in the garlic and ginger and cook for 1 minute until fragrant.

5. Add the soy sauce, rice vinegar, and sesame oil. Toss to coat the turkey and vegetables.

6. Add the cooked whole wheat noodles to the skillet and toss everything together until well combined.

7. Season the stir•fry with salt and pepper to taste. Serve the turkey and vegetable stir•fry with whole wheat noodles immediately.

The combination of lean protein, fiber•rich vegetables, and whole grains makes this a nutritious and filling meal that can be beneficial for women managing fatty liver disease.

65. Grilled shrimp with a mango avocado salsa

Ingredients:

Salsa:
• 1 ripe mango, diced
• 1 avocado, diced
• 1/4 cup diced red onion
• 1 jalapeño, seeded and minced
• 2 tbsp chopped fresh cilantro
• 1 tbsp lime juice
• Salt and pepper to taste

Shrimp:
• 1 lb large shrimp, peeled and deveined
• 1 tbsp olive oil
• 1 tsp chili powder
• 1/2 tsp garlic powder
• Salt and pepper to taste

Instructions:
1. Make the salsa: In a medium bowl, combine the diced mango, avocado, red onion, jalapeño, cilantro, and lime juice. Season with salt and pepper to taste. Set aside.

2. Prepare the shrimp: In a large bowl, toss the shrimp with the olive oil, chili powder, garlic powder, salt, and pepper.

3. Preheat a grill or grill pan over medium•high heat. Grill the shrimp for 2•3 minutes per side, until opaque and cooked through.

4. Serve the grilled shrimp immediately, topped with the mango avocado salsa.

This recipe is supportive for a fatty liver diet for women for a few reasons:

• Shrimp is a lean protein that is low in saturated fat, which is important for fatty liver disease.
• Mango and avocado are both nutrient•dense fruits that are high in fiber, vitamins, and antioxidants to support liver health.
• The olive oil provides healthy unsaturated fats.
• The dish is grilled, which is a healthy cooking method that doesn't require a lot of added oils or fats.

66. Quinoa and vegetable stuffed portobello mushrooms

Ingredients:

- 4 large portobello mushroom caps, stems removed and chopped
- 1 cup cooked quinoa
- 1 cup diced zucchini
- 1/2 cup diced red bell pepper
- 1/2 cup diced onion
- 2 cloves garlic, minced
- 2 tbsp chopped fresh basil
- 1 tbsp olive oil
- 1/4 cup crumbled feta cheese
- Salt and pepper to taste

Instructions:

1. Preheat the oven to 400°F. Arrange the portobello mushroom caps, gill•side up, on a baking sheet.

2. In a large skillet, heat the olive oil over medium heat. Add the chopped mushroom stems, zucchini, bell pepper, onion, and garlic. Sauté for 5•7 minutes until the vegetables are tender.

3. Remove the skillet from heat and stir in the cooked quinoa, fresh basil, salt, and pepper.

4. Spoon the quinoa and vegetable mixture evenly into the portobello mushroom caps.

5. Sprinkle the crumbled feta cheese over the top of the stuffed mushrooms.

6. Bake for 15•20 minutes, until the mushrooms are tender and the filling is hot.

7. Serve the quinoa and vegetable stuffed portobello mushrooms warm.

The combination of whole grains, vegetables, and a moderate amount of healthy fat makes this a nutritious and liver•friendly meal option. Enjoy!

67. Lentil and sweet potato curry with brown rice

Ingredients:

Curry:
• 1 cup dry brown or green lentils, rinsed
• 2 cups diced sweet potatoes
• 1 onion, diced
• 3 cloves garlic, minced
• 1 tbsp grated fresh ginger
• 2 tsp curry powder
• 1 tsp ground cumin
• 1 tsp ground coriander
• 1 (14 oz) can diced tomatoes
• 1 cup low•sodium vegetable broth
• 1 cup light coconut milk
• Salt and pepper to taste
• Chopped cilantro for garnish

Brown Rice:
• 1 cup uncooked brown rice
• 2 cups low•sodium vegetable or chicken broth

Instructions:

1. Cook the brown rice: In a medium saucepan, bring the 2 cups of broth to a boil. Add the brown rice, cover, reduce heat to low and simmer for 25•30 minutes until rice is tender. Fluff with a fork.

2. Make the curry: In a large pot or Dutch oven, sauté the onion in a splash of vegetable broth over medium heat for 5 minutes until translucent.

3. Add the garlic and ginger and cook for 1 minute until fragrant.

4. Stir in the curry powder, cumin, and coriander and cook for 1 minute.

5. Add the lentils, sweet potatoes, diced tomatoes, vegetable broth, and coconut milk. Bring to a simmer and cook for 20•25 minutes, until the lentils and sweet potatoes are very soft.

6. Season the curry with salt and pepper to taste. Serve the lentil and sweet potato curry over the cooked brown rice. Garnish with chopped cilantro.

The combination of fiber•rich lentils and vegetables, healthy fats, and whole grains makes this a great option for a fatty liver•friendly meal. Enjoy!

68. Spinach and feta stuffed chicken breasts with a side of quinoa

Ingredients:

Stuffed Chicken:
- 4 boneless, skinless chicken breasts
- 1 cup fresh spinach, chopped
- 1/2 cup crumbled feta cheese
- 1 clove garlic, minced
- 1 tbsp olive oil
- Salt and pepper to taste

Quinoa:
- 1 cup uncooked quinoa, rinsed
- 2 cups low•sodium chicken or vegetable broth

Instructions:

1. Preheat the oven to 400°F.

2. Prepare the quinoa: In a medium saucepan, bring the broth to a boil. Add the quinoa, cover, reduce heat to low and simmer for 15•20 minutes until quinoa is tender and liquid is absorbed.

3. Make the stuffed chicken: Use a sharp knife to cut a pocket into the side of each chicken breast.

4. In a small bowl, mix together the chopped spinach, feta cheese, and minced garlic.

5. Stuff each chicken breast with the spinach and feta mixture, being careful not to overstuff.

6. Place the stuffed chicken breasts in a baking dish and drizzle with the olive oil. Season with salt and pepper.

7. Bake the chicken for 25•30 minutes, until the chicken is cooked through and the internal temperature reaches 165°F. Serve the spinach and feta stuffed chicken breasts warm, alongside the cooked quinoa.

The combination of lean protein, fiber•rich vegetables and whole grains makes this a well•balanced and liver•friendly meal. Enjoy!

69. Baked salmon with roasted Brussels sprouts and sweet potatoes

Ingredients:
Roasted Vegetables:
• 1 lb Brussels sprouts, trimmed and halved
• 2 medium sweet potatoes, peeled and cubed
• 2 tbsp olive oil
• Salt and pepper to taste

Salmon:
• 4 (6 oz) salmon fillets
• 1 tbsp olive oil
• 1 tsp lemon zest
• 1 tsp dried dill
• Salt and pepper to taste

Instructions:

1. Preheat the oven to 400°F.

2. Prepare the roasted vegetables: In a large baking dish, toss the Brussels sprouts and sweet potato cubes with the 2 tbsp of olive oil. Season with salt and pepper. Roast for 25•30 minutes, stirring halfway, until vegetables are tender and lightly browned.

3. While the vegetables are roasting, prepare the salmon. Place the salmon fillets on a baking sheet. Drizzle with the 1 tbsp of olive oil and sprinkle with the lemon zest, dried dill, salt, and pepper.

4. Bake the salmon for 12•15 minutes, until it flakes easily with a fork. Serve the baked salmon fillets alongside the roasted Brussels sprouts and sweet potatoes.

This recipe is supportive for a fatty liver diet for women for a few reasons:

• Salmon is an excellent source of omega•3 fatty acids, which can help reduce inflammation.
• Brussels sprouts and sweet potatoes are high in fiber, vitamins, and antioxidants to support liver health.
• The dish is baked, not fried, keeping it light and healthy.

The combination of heart•healthy salmon, fiber•rich vegetables, and healthy cooking methods makes this a great option for a fatty liver•friendly meal. Enjoy!

70. Lentil and vegetable stir fry with tofu

Ingredients:

- 1 cup dry brown or green lentils, rinsed
- 1 block extra•firm tofu, pressed and cubed
- 2 tbsp sesame oil, divided
- 1 red bell pepper, sliced
- 1 cup broccoli florets
- 1 cup sliced mushrooms
- 2 cloves garlic, minced
- 1 tbsp grated fresh ginger
- 2 tbsp low•sodium soy sauce or tamari
- 1 tbsp rice vinegar
- Salt and pepper to taste
- Chopped green onions for garnish (optional)

Instructions:

1. Cook the lentils according to package instructions until tender. Drain and set aside.

2. In a large skillet or wok, heat 1 tbsp of the sesame oil over medium•high heat. Add the cubed tofu and cook for 3•4 minutes per side until lightly browned. Remove tofu from the pan and set aside.

3. In the same pan, heat the remaining 1 tbsp of sesame oil. Add the bell pepper, broccoli, and mushrooms. Stir•fry for 5•7 minutes until the vegetables are tender•crisp.

4. Stir in the garlic and ginger and cook for 1 minute until fragrant.

5. Add the cooked lentils, soy sauce, and rice vinegar. Toss everything together until well combined.

6. Gently fold the seared tofu back into the stir•fry.

7. Season the lentil and vegetable stir•fry with salt and pepper to taste.

8. Serve the stir•fry warm, garnished with chopped green onions if desired.

The combination of fiber•rich lentils, lean plant•based protein, and nutrient•dense vegetables makes this a nutritious and liver•friendly meal. Enjoy!

71. Turkey and black bean lettuce wraps with a side of brown rice

Ingredients:

Lettuce Wraps:
• 1 lb ground turkey
• 1 (15 oz) can black beans, rinsed and drained
• 1 cup diced bell pepper
• 1/2 cup diced onion
• 2 cloves garlic, minced
• 1 tsp ground cumin
• 1 tsp chili powder
• Salt and pepper to taste
• Bibb or romaine lettuce leaves for wrapping

Brown Rice:
• 1 cup uncooked brown rice
• 2 cups low•sodium chicken or vegetable broth

Instructions:

1. Cook the brown rice: In a medium saucepan, bring the broth to a boil. Add the brown rice, cover, reduce heat to low and simmer for 25•30 minutes until rice is tender.

2. Make the lettuce wraps: In a large skillet over medium•high heat, cook the ground turkey, breaking it up with a wooden spoon, until no longer pink, about 5•7 minutes.

3. Add the black beans, bell pepper, onion, garlic, cumin, and chili powder. Stir and cook for 5 minutes until the vegetables are tender.

4. Season the turkey and black bean mixture with salt and pepper to taste. To serve, spoon the turkey and black bean filling into the lettuce leaves. Serve with the cooked brown rice on the side.

This recipe is supportive for a fatty liver diet for women for a few reasons:

• Ground turkey is a lean protein that is low in saturated fat.
• Black beans are a great source of plant•based protein and fiber.
• The vegetables, including bell pepper and onion, are high in fiber, vitamins, and antioxidants.
• Brown rice is a whole grain that is high in fiber and nutrients.
• The dish is light and fresh, without any heavy sauces or fried elements

72. Greek yogurt parfait with granola and berries

Ingredients:

- 2 cups plain Greek yogurt
- 1 cup mixed berries (such as blueberries, raspberries, and/or strawberries)
- 1/2 cup homemade or store•bought granola
- 1 tbsp honey (optional)

Instructions:

1. In a parfait glass or bowl, layer the ingredients in the following order:
   - 1/2 cup Greek yogurt
   - 1/4 cup mixed berries
   - 2 tbsp granola
   - Repeat the layers
   - Top with the remaining 1/2 cup yogurt

2. If desired, drizzle 1 tbsp of honey over the top of the parfait.

3. Serve chilled.

This recipe is supportive for a fatty liver diet for women for a few reasons:

• Greek yogurt is an excellent source of protein, which is important for maintaining muscle mass and supporting overall health. It's also lower in fat compared to regular yogurt.

• Berries are high in fiber, vitamins, and antioxidants that can help support liver health. Blueberries, raspberries, and strawberries are all great options.

• Granola provides a crunchy texture and a source of complex carbohydrates and fiber. Look for a granola that is low in added sugars.

• Honey is a natural sweetener that can be used in moderation to add a touch of sweetness.

The combination of protein•rich Greek yogurt, fiber•filled berries, and complex carbohydrates from the granola makes this a nutrient•dense and satisfying snack or light meal that can be beneficial for women managing fatty liver disease. It's easy to prepare and provides a delicious way to incorporate more healthy foods into the diet.

73. Quinoa and black bean burgers with a side salad

Ingredients:

Burgers:
• 1 cup cooked quinoa
• 1 (15 oz) can black beans, rinsed and drained
• 1/2 cup rolled oats
• 1/4 cup diced onion
• 2 cloves garlic, minced
• 1 tsp ground cumin
• 1/2 tsp chili powder
• Salt and pepper to taste
• Whole wheat buns or lettuce wraps

Side Salad:
• 4 cups mixed greens
• 1/2 cup diced cucumber
• 1/4 cup diced tomatoes
• 2 tbsp crumbled feta cheese
• 1 tbsp olive oil
• 1 tbsp balsamic vinegar
• Salt and pepper to taste

Instructions:

1. In a large bowl, mash the black beans with a fork or potato masher. Stir in the cooked quinoa, rolled oats, onion, garlic, cumin, chili powder, salt, and pepper until well combined.

2. Form the mixture into 4•6 patties, about 1/2 inch thick.

3. Heat a large skillet over medium heat and cook the quinoa and black bean burgers for 3•4 minutes per side, until lightly browned.

4. Serve the burgers on whole wheat buns or in lettuce wraps, with the side salad.

For the side salad:
1. In a large bowl, combine the mixed greens, cucumber, tomatoes, and feta cheese.
2. Drizzle the olive oil and balsamic vinegar over the salad and toss to coat.
3. Season the salad with salt and pepper to taste.

The combination of lean protein, fiber•rich vegetables, and healthy fats makes this a well•balanced and liver•friendly meal. Enjoy!

74. Grilled chicken with roasted root vegetables and quinoa

Ingredients:

Roasted Vegetables:
• 1 lb carrots, peeled and
cut into 1•inch pieces
• 1 lb sweet potatoes,
peeled and cut into 1•inch cubes
• 1 red onion, cut into wedges
• 2 tbsp olive oil
• Salt and pepper to taste

Chicken:
• 4 boneless, skinless chicken breasts
• 1 tbsp olive oil
• 1 tsp dried thyme
• 1/2 tsp garlic powder
• Salt and pepper to taste

Quinoa:
• 1 cup uncooked quinoa, rinsed
• 2 cups low•sodium chicken or vegetable broth

Instructions:

1. Preheat the oven to 400°F.

2. Prepare the roasted vegetables: In a large baking dish, toss the carrots, sweet potatoes, and onion with the 2 tbsp of olive oil. Season with salt and pepper. Roast for 25•30 minutes, stirring halfway, until the vegetables are tender and lightly browned.

3. While the vegetables are roasting, prepare the quinoa. In a medium saucepan, bring the broth to a boil. Add the quinoa, cover, reduce heat to low and simmer for 15•20 minutes until quinoa is tender and liquid is absorbed.

4. Prepare the chicken: Brush the chicken breasts with the 1 tbsp of olive oil and season with the thyme, garlic powder, salt, and pepper.

5. Preheat a grill or grill pan over medium•high heat. Grill the chicken for 5•7 minutes per side, until cooked through and no longer pink in the center.

6. Serve the grilled chicken alongside the roasted root vegetables and cooked quinoa.

The combination of lean protein, fiber•rich vegetables, and nutrient•dense whole grains makes this a well•balanced and liver•friendly meal. Enjoy!

75. Tofu and vegetable curry with brown rice

Ingredients:
- 1 block of firm or extra•firm tofu, cubed
- 1 onion, diced
- 3 cloves garlic, minced
- 1 inch ginger, grated
- 1 bell pepper, diced
- 1 cup sliced mushrooms
- 1 cup chopped spinach or kale
- 1 can (13.5 oz) coconut milk
- 2 tbsp curry powder
- 1 tsp ground cumin
- 1 tsp ground coriander
- Salt and pepper to taste
- 1 cup cooked brown rice

Instructions:
1. In a large skillet or wok, sauté the onion, garlic, and ginger in a small amount of oil or broth over medium heat until fragrant and translucent.

2. Add the bell pepper, mushrooms, and tofu. Cook for 5•7 minutes, stirring occasionally, until the vegetables are tender.

3. Pour in the coconut milk and stir in the curry powder, cumin, and coriander. Bring to a simmer and let the sauce thicken for 5•10 minutes.

4. Stir in the spinach or kale and season with salt and pepper to taste.

5. Serve the curry over a bed of cooked brown rice.

This dish is supportive for a fatty liver diet as it is:
- High in plant•based protein from the tofu
- Rich in fiber and antioxidants from the vegetables
- Contains healthy fats from the coconut milk
- Uses whole grain brown rice as the base

76. Turkey and vegetable stir fry with quinoa

Ingredients:

- 1 lb ground turkey
- 2 cups mixed vegetables (such as broccoli, bell peppers, snap peas, mushrooms)
- 1 onion, diced
- 3 cloves garlic, minced
- 1 inch ginger, grated
- 2 tbsp low•sodium soy sauce or tamari
- 1 tbsp rice vinegar
- 1 tsp sesame oil
- 1 tsp cornstarch
- Salt and pepper to taste
- 1 cup cooked quinoa

Instructions:

1. In a large skillet or wok, cook the ground turkey over medium•high heat, breaking it up as it cooks, until browned and cooked through, about 5•7 minutes. Transfer the turkey to a plate.

2. In the same skillet, add a splash of broth or water and sauté the onion, garlic, and ginger for 2•3 minutes until fragrant.

3. Add the mixed vegetables and continue to stir•fry for 5•7 minutes until the vegetables are tender•crisp.

4. In a small bowl, whisk together the soy sauce, rice vinegar, sesame oil, and cornstarch.

5. Return the cooked turkey to the skillet and pour in the sauce mixture. Toss everything together and let the sauce thicken for 1•2 minutes.

6. Serve the turkey and vegetable stir•fry over a bed of cooked quinoa.

This dish is supportive for a fatty liver diet as it is:
- High in lean protein from the turkey
- Rich in fiber and antioxidants from the vegetables
- Contains whole grain quinoa as the base
- Uses a light sauce with minimal added sugars

The combination of nutrients can help support liver health and function. Enjoy this flavorful and nourishing stir•fry!

77. Lentil and vegetable stuffed bell peppers

Ingredients:
- 4 bell peppers, halved and seeded
- 1 cup cooked brown or green lentils
- 1 cup diced tomatoes
- 1/2 cup diced onion
- 2 cloves garlic, minced
- 1 cup chopped spinach or kale
- 1 tsp ground cumin
- 1 tsp dried oregano
- 1/4 tsp red pepper flakes (optional)
- Salt and pepper to taste
- 1/4 cup crumbled feta cheese (optional)

Instructions:
1. Preheat the oven to 375°F. Place the bell pepper halves in a baking dish and set aside.

2. In a skillet over medium heat, sauté the onion and garlic until translucent, about 3•5 minutes.

3. Add the lentils, diced tomatoes, spinach/kale, cumin, oregano, and red pepper flakes (if using). Season with salt and pepper.

4. Spoon the lentil and vegetable mixture into the bell pepper halves, packing it in tightly.

5. Bake the stuffed peppers for 25•30 minutes, until the peppers are tender.

6. Remove from the oven and top with crumbled feta cheese, if desired.

This dish is supportive for a fatty liver diet as it is:
- High in plant•based protein and fiber from the lentils
- Rich in antioxidants and vitamins from the bell peppers and greens
- Contains healthy fats from the optional feta cheese
- Uses whole food ingredients without added sugars or unhealthy fats

The combination of nutrients can help support liver health and function. Enjoy these flavorful and nourishing stuffed bell peppers!

78. Baked cod with a lemon herb quinoa salad

Ingredients:

Baked Cod:
• 4 cod fillets (about 4•6 oz each)
• 2 tbsp olive oil
• 1 tsp lemon zest
• 1 tbsp lemon juice
• 2 cloves garlic, minced
• Salt and pepper to taste

Lemon Herb Quinoa Salad:
• 1 cup cooked quinoa
• 1 cup diced cucumber
• 1/2 cup diced tomatoes
• 1/4 cup chopped parsley
• 2 tbsp chopped fresh dill
• 2 tbsp lemon juice
• 1 tbsp olive oil
• Salt and pepper to taste

Instructions:

1. Preheat the oven to 400°F. Line a baking sheet with parchment paper.

2. In a small bowl, mix together the olive oil, lemon zest, lemon juice, garlic, salt, and pepper. Place the cod fillets on the prepared baking sheet and brush the top with the lemon•garlic mixture.

3. Bake the cod for 12•15 minutes, or until it flakes easily with a fork.

4. While the cod is baking, prepare the quinoa salad. In a medium bowl, combine the cooked quinoa, cucumber, tomatoes, parsley, dill, lemon juice, and olive oil. Season with salt and pepper.

5. Serve the baked cod fillets warm, topped with the lemon herb quinoa salad.

This dish is supportive for a fatty liver diet as it is:
• High in lean protein from the cod
• Rich in fiber and antioxidants from the quinoa, vegetables, and herbs
• Contains healthy fats from the olive oil
• Uses minimal added sugars or unhealthy ingredients

79. Spinach and feta stuffed portobello mushrooms

Ingredients:
• 4 large portobello mushroom caps, stems removed and chopped
• 2 cups fresh spinach, chopped
• 1/2 cup crumbled feta cheese
• 2 cloves garlic, minced
• 1 tbsp olive oil
• 1/4 tsp dried oregano
• Salt and pepper to taste

Instructions:
1. Preheat the oven to 400°F. Lightly grease a baking sheet or line it with parchment paper.

2. Gently clean the portobello mushroom caps with a damp paper towel. Remove the stems and chop them.

3. In a skillet over medium heat, sauté the chopped mushroom stems and garlic in the olive oil for 2•3 minutes until fragrant.

4. Add the chopped spinach and continue cooking for 2•3 minutes until the spinach is wilted.

5. Remove the skillet from heat and stir in the crumbled feta cheese, oregano, salt, and pepper.

6. Spoon the spinach and feta mixture evenly into the portobello mushroom caps, packing it in gently.

7. Place the stuffed mushrooms on the prepared baking sheet.

8. Bake for 15•20 minutes, until the mushrooms are tender and the filling is hot.

9. Serve the stuffed portobello mushrooms warm.

This dish is supportive for a fatty liver diet as it is:
• High in fiber and antioxidants from the portobello mushrooms and spinach

• Contains healthy fats from the olive oil and feta cheese

• Uses whole food ingredients without added sugars or unhealthy fats

80. Grilled shrimp with a mango salsa and quinoa

Ingredients:

Grilled Shrimp:
- 1 lb large shrimp, peeled and deveined
- 2 tbsp olive oil
- 1 tsp chili powder
- 1 tsp garlic powder
- Salt and pepper to taste

Quinoa:
- 1 cup cooked quinoa

Mango Salsa:
- 1 ripe mango, diced
- 1/2 red onion, diced
- 1 jalapeño, seeded and minced
- 1/4 cup chopped cilantro
- 2 tbsp lime juice
- 1 tbsp olive oil
- Salt and pepper to taste

Instructions:

1. Preheat grill or grill pan to medium·high heat.

2. In a bowl, toss the shrimp with the olive oil, chili powder, garlic powder, salt, and pepper.

3. Grill the shrimp for 2·3 minutes per side, until opaque and cooked through. Set aside.

4. In a separate bowl, combine all the mango salsa ingredients and mix well. Season with salt and pepper.

5. Serve the grilled shrimp over a bed of cooked quinoa, topped with the mango salsa.

This dish is supportive for a fatty liver diet as it is:

- High in lean protein from the shrimp

- Rich in fiber and antioxidants from the quinoa, mango, and vegetables

- Contains healthy fats from the olive oil

- Uses minimal added sugars or unhealthy ingredients

The combination of nutrients can help support liver health and function. Enjoy this flavorful and nourishing grilled shrimp dish!

81. Lentil and vegetable soup with whole wheat bread

Ingredients:

Soup:
• 1 cup brown or green lentils, rinsed
• 1 onion, diced
• 3 carrots, peeled and diced
• 3 celery stalks, diced
• 3 cloves garlic, minced
• 1 tsp ground cumin
• 1 tsp dried thyme
• 4 cups low•sodium vegetable or chicken broth
• 1 (14.5 oz) can diced tomatoes
• Salt and pepper to taste

Whole Wheat Bread:• 1 loaf whole wheat bread

Instructions:

1. In a large pot, sauté the onion, carrots, celery, and garlic in a small amount of broth or olive oil over medium heat for 5•7 minutes until softened.

2. Add the lentils, cumin, thyme, broth, and diced tomatoes. Bring to a boil, then reduce heat and simmer for 20•25 minutes, until the lentils are tender.

3. Season the soup with salt and pepper to taste.

4. Serve the lentil and vegetable soup warm, with slices of whole wheat bread on the side.

This meal is supportive for a fatty liver diet as it is:

• High in plant•based protein and fiber from the lentils

• Rich in antioxidants and vitamins from the vegetables

• Contains whole grains from the whole wheat bread

• Uses low•sodium broth and minimal added fats or sugars

The combination of nutrients can help support liver health and function. Enjoy this nourishing and comforting soup and bread pairing!

82. Turkey and vegetable stir fry with brown rice noodles

Ingredients:

• 8 oz brown rice noodles
• 1 lb ground turkey
• 2 cups mixed vegetables (such as broccoli, bell peppers, snap peas, mushrooms)
• 1 onion, sliced
• 3 cloves garlic, minced
• 1 inch ginger, grated
• 2 tbsp low•sodium soy sauce or tamari
• 1 tbsp rice vinegar
• 1 tsp sesame oil
• 1 tsp cornstarch
• Salt and pepper to taste

Instructions:

1. Cook the brown rice noodles according to package instructions. Drain and set aside.

2. In a large skillet or wok, cook the ground turkey over medium•high heat, breaking it up as it cooks, until browned and cooked through, about 5•7 minutes. Transfer the turkey to a plate.

3. In the same skillet, add a splash of broth or water and sauté the onion, garlic, and ginger for 2•3 minutes until fragrant.

4. Add the mixed vegetables and continue to stir•fry for 5•7 minutes until the vegetables are tender•crisp.

5. In a small bowl, whisk together the soy sauce, rice vinegar, sesame oil, and cornstarch.

6. Return the cooked turkey to the skillet and pour in the sauce mixture. Toss everything together and let the sauce thicken for 1•2 minutes.

7. Add the cooked brown rice noodles to the skillet and toss to combine. Serve the turkey and vegetable stir•fry with brown rice noodles warm.

This dish is supportive for a fatty liver diet as it is:
• High in lean protein from the turkey
• Rich in fiber and antioxidants from the vegetables and brown rice noodles
• Contains healthy fats from the sesame oil
• Uses a light sauce with minimal added sugars

83. Quinoa and black bean stuffed bell peppers

Ingredients:

• 4 bell peppers, halved and seeded
• 1 cup cooked quinoa
• 1 (15 oz) can black beans, rinsed and drained
• 1 cup diced tomatoes
• 1/2 cup diced onion
• 2 cloves garlic, minced
• 1 tsp ground cumin
• 1 tsp dried oregano
• 1/4 tsp chili powder
• Salt and pepper to taste
• 1/4 cup shredded cheddar or Monterey Jack cheese (optional)

Instructions:

1. Preheat the oven to 375°F. Place the bell pepper halves in a baking dish and set aside.

2. In a skillet over medium heat, sauté the onion and garlic until translucent, about 3•5 minutes.

3. Add the cooked quinoa, black beans, diced tomatoes, cumin, oregano, chili powder, salt, and pepper. Stir to combine.

4. Spoon the quinoa and black bean mixture evenly into the bell pepper halves, packing it in tightly.

5. If using, sprinkle the shredded cheese over the top of the stuffed peppers.

6. Bake the stuffed peppers for 25•30 minutes, until the peppers are tender. Remove from the oven and serve warm.

This dish is supportive for a fatty liver diet as it is:
• High in plant•based protein and fiber from the quinoa and black beans
• Rich in antioxidants and vitamins from the bell peppers and tomatoes
• Contains minimal added fats or sugars
• Uses whole food ingredients

The combination of nutrients can help support liver health and function. Enjoy these flavorful and nourishing stuffed bell peppers!

84. Baked salmon with roasted vegetables and quinoa

Ingredients:

Salmon:
• 4 salmon fillets (4•6 oz each)
• 1 tbsp olive oil
• 1 tsp lemon zest
• 1 tbsp lemon juice
• Salt and pepper to taste

Roasted Vegetables:
• 2 cups mixed vegetables (such as broccoli, bell peppers, zucchini, onions)
• 1 tbsp olive oil
• 1 tsp dried thyme
• Salt and pepper to taste

Quinoa:• 1 cup cooked quinoa

Instructions:

1. Preheat the oven to 400°F. Line a baking sheet with parchment paper.

2. In a small bowl, mix together the olive oil, lemon zest, lemon juice, salt, and pepper. Place the salmon fillets on the prepared baking sheet and brush the top with the lemon•herb mixture.

3. Toss the mixed vegetables with the olive oil, thyme, salt, and pepper. Spread the vegetables on a separate baking sheet.

4. Bake the salmon and vegetables for 15•20 minutes, until the salmon is cooked through and the vegetables are tender.

5. Serve the baked salmon over a bed of cooked quinoa, topped with the roasted vegetables.

This dish is supportive for a fatty liver diet as it is:
• High in lean protein from the salmon
• Rich in fiber, antioxidants, and healthy fats from the quinoa, vegetables, and olive oil
• Uses minimal added sugars or unhealthy ingredients

The combination of nutrients can help support liver health and function. Enjoy this delicious and nourishing salmon, vegetable, and quinoa meal!

85. Lentil and vegetable curry with brown rice

Ingredients:

• 1 cup brown or green lentils, rinsed
• 1 onion, diced
• 3 cloves garlic, minced
• 1 inch ginger, grated
• 2 cups mixed vegetables (such as cauliflower, spinach, bell peppers, peas)
• 1 can (13.5 oz) coconut milk
• 2 tbsp curry powder
• 1 tsp ground cumin
• 1 tsp ground coriander
• Salt and pepper to taste
• 1 cup cooked brown rice

Instructions:

1. In a large pot, bring 3 cups of water to a boil. Add the lentils, reduce heat, and simmer for 15•20 minutes until tender. Drain and set aside.

2. In the same pot, sauté the onion, garlic, and ginger in a small amount of oil or broth over medium heat until fragrant and translucent.

3. Add the mixed vegetables and continue cooking for 5•7 minutes until the vegetables are tender.

4. Pour in the coconut milk and stir in the curry powder, cumin, and coriander. Bring to a simmer and let the sauce thicken for 5•10 minutes.

5. Stir the cooked lentils into the curry. Season with salt and pepper to taste.

6. Serve the lentil and vegetable curry over a bed of cooked brown rice.

This dish is supportive for a fatty liver diet as it is:
• High in plant•based protein and fiber from the lentils
• Rich in antioxidants and vitamins from the vegetables
• Contains healthy fats from the coconut milk
• Uses whole grain brown rice as the base

The combination of nutrients can help support liver health and function. Enjoy this flavorful and nourishing curry!

86. Grilled chicken with steamed broccoli and quinoa

Ingredients:

Grilled Chicken:
• 4 boneless, skinless chicken breasts
• 1 tbsp olive oil
• 1 tsp garlic powder
• 1 tsp dried oregano
• Salt and pepper to taste

Steamed Broccoli:
• 2 cups broccoli florets
• 1/4 cup water

Quinoa: 1 cup cooked quinoa

Instructions:

1. Preheat grill or grill pan to medium•high heat.

2. In a shallow dish, rub the chicken breasts with the olive oil, garlic powder, oregano, salt, and pepper.

3. Grill the chicken for 5•7 minutes per side, or until cooked through and no longer pink in the center.

4. While the chicken is grilling, place the broccoli florets and water in a steamer basket. Steam the broccoli for 5•7 minutes, until tender•crisp.

5. Prepare the quinoa according to package instructions.

6. Serve the grilled chicken breast over a bed of cooked quinoa, with the steamed broccoli on the side.

This dish is supportive for a fatty liver diet as it is:
• High in lean protein from the grilled chicken
• Rich in fiber, antioxidants, and vitamins from the broccoli and quinoa
• Contains healthy fats from the olive oil
• Uses minimal added sugars or unhealthy ingredients

The combination of nutrients can help support liver health and function. Enjoy this simple and nourishing grilled chicken, broccoli, and quinoa meal!

87. Tofu and vegetable stir fry with brown rice

Ingredients:

• 1 block (14 oz) extra•firm tofu, cubed
• 2 cups mixed vegetables (such as broccoli, bell peppers, snap peas, mushrooms)
• 1 onion, sliced
• 3 cloves garlic, minced
• 1 inch ginger, grated
• 2 tbsp low•sodium soy sauce or tamari
• 1 tbsp rice vinegar
• 1 tsp sesame oil
• 1 tsp cornstarch
• Salt and pepper to taste
• 1 cup cooked brown rice

Instructions:

1. In a large skillet or wok, heat a small amount of oil or broth over medium•high heat. Add the tofu cubes and cook for 5•7 minutes, turning occasionally, until lightly browned on all sides. Transfer the tofu to a plate.

2. In the same skillet, add the onion, garlic, and ginger. Sauté for 2•3 minutes until fragrant.

3. Add the mixed vegetables and continue to stir•fry for 5•7 minutes until the vegetables are tender•crisp.

4. In a small bowl, whisk together the soy sauce, rice vinegar, sesame oil, and cornstarch.

5. Return the cooked tofu to the skillet and pour in the sauce mixture. Toss everything together and let the sauce thicken for 1•2 minutes.

6. Serve the tofu and vegetable stir•fry over a bed of cooked brown rice.

This dish is supportive for a fatty liver diet as it is:
• High in plant•based protein from the tofu
• Rich in fiber and antioxidants from the vegetables and brown rice
• Contains healthy fats from the sesame oil
• Uses a light sauce with minimal added sugars

The combination of nutrients can help support liver health and function. Enjoy this flavorful and nourishing stir•fry!

88. Turkey and black bean lettuce wraps with a side of quinoa

Ingredients:

Lettuce Wraps:
• 1 lb ground turkey
• 1 (15 oz) can black beans, rinsed and drained
• 1 onion, diced
• 2 cloves garlic, minced
• 1 tsp ground cumin
• 1 tsp chili powder
• Salt and pepper to taste
• 8•10 large lettuce leaves (such as romaine or bibb)

Quinoa:• 1 cup cooked quinoa

Instructions:

1. In a large skillet over medium heat, cook the ground turkey, breaking it up as it cooks, until browned and cooked through, about 5•7 minutes.

2. Add the diced onion and minced garlic to the skillet. Cook for 2•3 minutes until the onion is translucent.

3. Stir in the black beans, cumin, chili powder, salt, and pepper. Cook for an additional 2•3 minutes to heat through.

4. Prepare the quinoa according to package instructions.

5. To assemble the lettuce wraps, place a couple tablespoons of the turkey and black bean mixture into the center of a lettuce leaf. Fold or wrap the lettuce around the filling.

6. Serve the turkey and black bean lettuce wraps with a side of cooked quinoa.

This dish is supportive for a fatty liver diet as it is:
• High in lean protein from the turkey and black beans
• Rich in fiber and antioxidants from the lettuce, quinoa, and vegetables
• Contains minimal added fats or sugars
• Uses whole food ingredients

The combination of nutrients can help support liver health and function. Enjoy these flavorful and nourishing turkey and black bean lettuce wraps with quinoa!

89. Lentil and sweet potato curry with quinoa

Ingredients:

• 1 cup brown or green lentils, rinsed
• 2 cups diced sweet potatoes
• 1 onion, diced
• 3 cloves garlic, minced
• 1 inch ginger, grated
• 2 tsp curry powder
• 1 tsp ground cumin
• 1 tsp ground coriander
• 1 can (13.5 oz) coconut milk
• 1 cup vegetable or chicken broth
• Salt and pepper to taste
• 1 cup cooked quinoa

Instructions:

1. In a large pot, bring 3 cups of water to a boil. Add the lentils, reduce heat, and simmer for 15•20 minutes until tender. Drain and set aside.

2. In the same pot, sauté the onion, garlic, and ginger in a small amount of oil or broth over medium heat until fragrant and translucent.

3. Add the diced sweet potatoes, curry powder, cumin, and coriander. Stir to coat the vegetables in the spices.

4. Pour in the coconut milk and broth. Bring to a simmer and let the sweet potatoes cook for 15•20 minutes until tender.

5. Stir the cooked lentils into the curry. Season with salt and pepper to taste.

6. Serve the lentil and sweet potato curry over a bed of cooked quinoa.

This dish is supportive for a fatty liver diet as it is:
• High in plant•based protein and fiber from the lentils
• Rich in antioxidants and vitamins from the sweet potatoes and quinoa
• Contains healthy fats from the coconut milk
• Uses minimal added sugars or unhealthy ingredients

The combination of nutrients can help support liver health and function. Enjoy this flavorful and nourishing curry!

90. Spinach and feta stuffed chicken breasts with a side salad

Ingredients:

Stuffed Chicken:
• 4 boneless, skinless chicken breasts
• 1 cup fresh spinach, chopped
• 1/2 cup crumbled feta cheese
• 2 cloves garlic, minced
• 1 tbsp olive oil
• Salt and pepper to taste

Side Salad:
• 4 cups mixed greens
• 1 cup cherry tomatoes, halved
• 1/2 cucumber, sliced
• 2 tbsp olive oil
• 1 tbsp balsamic vinegar
• Salt and pepper to taste

Instructions:

1. Preheat the oven to 375°F. Lightly grease a baking dish.

2. In a bowl, mix together the chopped spinach, feta cheese, and minced garlic.

3. Slice a pocket into the side of each chicken breast. Stuff the spinach and feta mixture evenly into the pockets.

4. Place the stuffed chicken breasts in the prepared baking dish. Drizzle with the olive oil and season with salt and pepper.

5. Bake the stuffed chicken for 25•30 minutes, until the chicken is cooked through and the internal temperature reaches 165°F.

6. While the chicken is baking, prepare the side salad. In a large bowl, combine the mixed greens, cherry tomatoes, and cucumber slices.

7. Drizzle the salad with the olive oil and balsamic vinegar. Season with salt and pepper.

8. Serve the spinach and feta stuffed chicken breasts with the side salad.

This dish is supportive for a fatty liver diet as it is:
• High in lean protein from the chicken
• Rich in fiber, antioxidants, and vitamins from the spinach, greens, and vegetables
• Contains healthy fats from the olive oil and feta cheese
• Uses minimal added sugars or unhealthy ingredients

The combination of nutrients can help support liver health and function. Enjoy this delicious and nourishing stuffed chicken and salad meal!

91. Baked cod with roasted Brussels sprouts and sweet potatoes

Ingredients:

Baked Cod:
• 4 cod fillets (4•6 oz each)
• 1 tbsp olive oil
• 1 tsp lemon zest
• 1 tbsp lemon juice
• Salt and pepper to taste

Roasted Vegetables:
• 2 cups Brussels sprouts, trimmed and halved
• 2 cups cubed sweet potatoes
• 1 tbsp olive oil
• 1 tsp dried thyme
• Salt and pepper to taste

Instructions:

1. Preheat the oven to 400°F. Line two baking sheets with parchment paper.

2. In a small bowl, mix together the olive oil, lemon zest, lemon juice, salt, and pepper. Place the cod fillets on one of the prepared baking sheets and brush the top with the lemon•herb mixture.

3. Toss the Brussels sprouts and sweet potato cubes with the olive oil, thyme, salt, and pepper. Spread the vegetables on the second baking sheet.

4. Bake the cod and vegetables for 15•20 minutes, until the cod is cooked through and the vegetables are tender.

5. Serve the baked cod fillets with the roasted Brussels sprouts and sweet potatoes.

This dish is supportive for a fatty liver diet as it is:
• High in lean protein from the cod
• Rich in fiber, antioxidants, and vitamins from the Brussels sprouts and sweet potatoes
• Contains healthy fats from the olive oil
• Uses minimal added sugars or unhealthy ingredients

The combination of nutrients can help support liver health and function. Enjoy this delicious and nourishing baked cod and roasted vegetable meal!

92. Lentil and vegetable stir fry with tofu

Ingredients:

- 1 cup brown or green lentils, rinsed
- 1 block (14 oz) extra•firm tofu, cubed
- 2 cups mixed vegetables (such as broccoli, bell peppers, snap peas, mushrooms)
- 1 onion, sliced
- 3 cloves garlic, minced
- 1 inch ginger, grated
- 2 tbsp low•sodium soy sauce or tamari
- 1 tbsp rice vinegar
- 1 tsp sesame oil
- 1 tsp cornstarch
- Salt and pepper to taste

Instructions:

1. In a large pot, bring 3 cups of water to a boil. Add the lentils, reduce heat, and simmer for 15•20 minutes until tender. Drain and set aside.

2. In a large skillet or wok, heat a small amount of oil or broth over medium•high heat. Add the tofu cubes and cook for 5•7 minutes, turning occasionally, until lightly browned on all sides. Transfer the tofu to a plate.

3. In the same skillet, add the onion, garlic, and ginger. Sauté for 2•3 minutes until fragrant.

4. Add the mixed vegetables and continue to stir•fry for 5•7 minutes until the vegetables are tender•crisp.

5. In a small bowl, whisk together the soy sauce, rice vinegar, sesame oil, and cornstarch.

6. Return the cooked lentils and tofu to the skillet. Pour in the sauce mixture and toss everything together. Let the sauce thicken for 1•2 minutes.

7. Serve the lentil and vegetable stir•fry warm.

This dish is supportive for a fatty liver diet as it is:
- High in plant•based protein from the lentils and tofu
- Rich in fiber and antioxidants from the vegetables
- Contains healthy fats from the sesame oil
- Uses a light sauce with minimal added sugars

93. Turkey and vegetable lettuce wraps with a side of brown rice

Ingredients:

Lettuce Wraps:
• 1 lb ground turkey
• 1 cup diced mixed vegetables (such as bell peppers, mushrooms, carrots)
• 1 onion, diced
• 2 cloves garlic, minced
• 1 tsp ground cumin
• 1 tsp chili powder
• Salt and pepper to taste
• 8•10 large lettuce leaves (such as romaine or bibb)

Brown Rice: • 1 cup cooked brown rice

Instructions:

1. In a large skillet over medium heat, cook the ground turkey, breaking it up as it cooks, until browned and cooked through, about 5•7 minutes.

2. Add the diced vegetables, onion, and minced garlic to the skillet. Cook for 5•7 minutes until the vegetables are tender.

3. Stir in the cumin, chili powder, salt, and pepper. Cook for an additional 2•3 minutes.

4. Prepare the brown rice according to package instructions.

5. To assemble the lettuce wraps, place a couple tablespoons of the turkey and vegetable mixture into the center of a lettuce leaf. Fold or wrap the lettuce around the filling.

6. Serve the turkey and vegetable lettuce wraps with a side of cooked brown rice.

This dish is supportive for a fatty liver diet as it is:
• High in lean protein from the turkey
• Rich in fiber and antioxidants from the lettuce, vegetables, and brown rice
• Contains minimal added fats or sugars
• Uses whole food ingredients

The combination of nutrients can help support liver health and function. Enjoy these flavorful and nourishing turkey and vegetable lettuce wraps with a side of brown rice!

94. Greek yogurt parfait with granola and mixed berries

Ingredients:

- 2 cups plain Greek yogurt
- 1 cup mixed berries (such as blueberries, raspberries, blackberries)
- 1 cup homemade or store•bought granola (look for low•sugar varieties)
- 1 tbsp honey (optional)

Instructions:

1. In a parfait glass or bowl, layer the ingredients in the following order:
   - 1/2 cup Greek yogurt
   - 1/4 cup mixed berries
   - 1/4 cup granola
   - Repeat the layers

2. If desired, drizzle 1 tbsp of honey over the top of the parfait.

3. Serve chilled.

This parfait is supportive for a fatty liver diet as it is:

- High in protein from the Greek yogurt

- Rich in fiber and antioxidants from the berries and granola

- Contains minimal added sugars (the honey is optional)

- Uses whole food ingredients

The combination of nutrients can help support liver health and function. The Greek yogurt provides a good source of probiotics, which can also be beneficial for liver health. Enjoy this delicious and nutritious parfait!

95. Quinoa and black bean burgers with a side of sweet potato fries

Ingredients:

Quinoa and Black Bean Burgers:
• 1 cup cooked quinoa
• 1 (15 oz) can black beans, rinsed and drained
• 1/2 cup diced onion
• 2 cloves garlic, minced
• 1 tsp ground cumin
• 1 tsp chili powder
• 1/4 cup whole wheat breadcrumbs
• Salt and pepper to taste

Sweet Potato Fries:
• 2 medium sweet potatoes, peeled and cut into fry•shaped pieces
• 1 tbsp olive oil
• 1 tsp paprika
• Salt and pepper to taste

Instructions:

Quinoa and Black Bean Burgers:
1. In a large bowl, mash the black beans with a fork or potato masher.
2. Add the cooked quinoa, diced onion, garlic, cumin, chili powder, breadcrumbs, salt, and pepper. Mix well until fully combined.
3. Form the mixture into 4•6 patties.
4. Heat a small amount of oil in a skillet over medium heat. Cook the patties for 3•4 minutes per side, until lightly browned.

Sweet Potato Fries:
1. Preheat the oven to 400°F. Line a baking sheet with parchment paper.
2. Toss the sweet potato fries with the olive oil, paprika, salt, and pepper.
3. Spread the fries in a single layer on the prepared baking sheet.
4. Bake for 20•25 minutes, flipping halfway, until the fries are crispy.

Serve the quinoa and black bean burgers with the baked sweet potato fries.

This meal is supportive for a fatty liver diet as it is:
• High in plant•based protein and fiber from the quinoa and black beans
• Rich in antioxidants and vitamins from the sweet potatoes
• Contains healthy fats from the olive oil
• Uses whole food ingredients without added sugars

96. Grilled chicken with roasted root vegetables and quinoa

Ingredients:

Grilled Chicken:
- 4 boneless, skinless chicken breasts
- 1 tbsp olive oil
- 1 tsp garlic powder
- 1 tsp dried oregano
- Salt and pepper to taste

Roasted Root Vegetables:
- 2 cups cubed sweet potatoes
- 2 cups cubed beets
- 1 cup cubed carrots
- 1 tbsp olive oil
- 1 tsp dried thyme
- Salt and pepper to taste

Quinoa:
- 1 cup cooked quinoa

Instructions:

1. Preheat grill or grill pan to medium-high heat.

2. In a shallow dish, rub the chicken breasts with the olive oil, garlic powder, oregano, salt, and pepper.

3. Grill the chicken for 5-7 minutes per side, or until cooked through and no longer pink in the center.

4. Preheat the oven to 400°F. Line a baking sheet with parchment paper.

5. Toss the cubed sweet potatoes, beets, and carrots with the olive oil, thyme, salt, and pepper. Spread the vegetables in a single layer on the prepared baking sheet.

6. Roast the vegetables for 20-25 minutes, until tender and lightly browned.

7. Prepare the quinoa according to package instructions.

8. Serve the grilled chicken breast over a bed of cooked quinoa, with the roasted root vegetables on the side.

The combination of nutrients can help support liver health and function. Enjoy this nourishing and flavorful grilled chicken, roasted vegetable, and quinoa meal!

97. Tofu and vegetable curry with quinoa

Ingredients:
- 1 block (14 oz) extra•firm tofu, cubed
- 1 onion, diced
- 3 cloves garlic, minced
- 1 inch ginger, grated
- 2 cups mixed vegetables (such as cauliflower, spinach, bell peppers, peas)
- 1 can (13.5 oz) coconut milk
- 2 tbsp curry powder
- 1 tsp ground cumin
- 1 tsp ground coriander
- Salt and pepper to taste
- 1 cup cooked quinoa

Instructions:
1. In a large skillet or wok, heat a small amount of oil or broth over medium•high heat. Add the tofu cubes and cook for 5•7 minutes, turning occasionally, until lightly browned on all sides. Transfer the tofu to a plate.

2. In the same skillet, sauté the onion, garlic, and ginger until fragrant and translucent, about 2•3 minutes.

3. Add the mixed vegetables and continue cooking for 5•7 minutes until the vegetables are tender.

4. Pour in the coconut milk and stir in the curry powder, cumin, and coriander. Bring to a simmer and let the sauce thicken for 5•10 minutes.

5. Return the cooked tofu to the skillet and gently toss to combine. Season with salt and pepper to taste. Serve the tofu and vegetable curry over a bed of cooked quinoa.

This dish is supportive for a fatty liver diet as it is:
- High in plant•based protein from the tofu
- Rich in fiber, antioxidants, and vitamins from the vegetables and quinoa
- Contains healthy fats from the coconut milk
- Uses minimal added sugars or unhealthy ingredients

The combination of nutrients can help support liver health and function. Enjoy this flavorful and nourishing tofu and vegetable curry with quinoa!

98. Turkey and vegetable stir fry with soba noodles

Ingredients:

- 8 oz soba noodles
- 1 lb ground turkey
- 2 cups mixed vegetables (such as broccoli, bell peppers, snap peas, mushrooms)
- 1 onion, sliced
- 3 cloves garlic, minced
- 1 inch ginger, grated
- 2 tbsp low·sodium soy sauce or tamari
- 1 tbsp rice vinegar
- 1 tsp sesame oil
- 1 tsp cornstarch
- Salt and pepper to taste

Instructions:

1. Cook the soba noodles according to package instructions. Drain and set aside.

2. In a large skillet or wok, cook the ground turkey over medium·high heat, breaking it up as it cooks, until browned and cooked through, about 5·7 minutes. Transfer the turkey to a plate.

3. In the same skillet, add a splash of broth or water and sauté the onion, garlic, and ginger for 2·3 minutes until fragrant.

4. Add the mixed vegetables and continue to stir·fry for 5·7 minutes until the vegetables are tender·crisp.

5. In a small bowl, whisk together the soy sauce, rice vinegar, sesame oil, and cornstarch.

6. Return the cooked turkey to the skillet and pour in the sauce mixture. Toss everything together and let the sauce thicken for 1·2 minutes.

7. Add the cooked soba noodles to the skillet and toss to combine. Serve the turkey and vegetable stir·fry with soba noodles warm.

This dish is supportive for a fatty liver diet as it is:
- High in lean protein from the turkey
- Rich in fiber and antioxidants from the vegetables and soba noodles
- Contains healthy fats from the sesame oil
- Uses a light sauce with minimal added sugars

99. Lentil and vegetable stuffed bell peppers

Ingredients:

• 4 bell peppers, halved and seeded
• 1 cup cooked brown or green lentils
• 1 cup diced tomatoes
• 1/2 cup diced onion
• 2 cloves garlic, minced
• 1 cup chopped spinach or kale
• 1 tsp ground cumin
• 1 tsp dried oregano
• 1/4 tsp red pepper flakes (optional)
• Salt and pepper to taste
• 1/4 cup crumbled feta cheese (optional)

Instructions:

1. Preheat the oven to 375°F. Place the bell pepper halves in a baking dish and set aside.

2. In a skillet over medium heat, sauté the onion and garlic until translucent, about 3-5 minutes.

3. Add the lentils, diced tomatoes, spinach/kale, cumin, oregano, and red pepper flakes (if using). Season with salt and pepper.

4. Spoon the lentil and vegetable mixture into the bell pepper halves, packing it in tightly.

5. Bake the stuffed peppers for 25-30 minutes, until the peppers are tender.

6. Remove from the oven and top with crumbled feta cheese, if desired.

This dish is supportive for a fatty liver diet as it is:
• High in plant-based protein and fiber from the lentils
• Rich in antioxidants and vitamins from the bell peppers and greens
• Contains healthy fats from the optional feta cheese
• Uses whole food ingredients without added sugars or unhealthy fats

The combination of nutrients can help support liver health and function. Enjoy these flavorful and nourishing stuffed bell peppers!

100. Baked salmon with a lemon herb quinoa salad

Ingredients:

Baked Salmon:
• 4 salmon fillets (about 4•6 oz each)
• 2 tbsp olive oil
• 1 tsp lemon zest
• 1 tbsp lemon juice
• 2 cloves garlic, minced
• Salt and pepper to taste

Lemon Herb Quinoa Salad:
• 1 cup cooked quinoa
• 1 cup diced cucumber
• 1/2 cup diced tomatoes
• 1/4 cup chopped parsley
• 2 tbsp chopped fresh dill
• 2 tbsp lemon juice
• 1 tbsp olive oil
• Salt and pepper to taste

Instructions:

1. Preheat the oven to 400°F. Line a baking sheet with parchment paper.

2. In a small bowl, mix together the olive oil, lemon zest, lemon juice, garlic, salt, and pepper. Place the salmon fillets on the prepared baking sheet and brush the top with the lemon•garlic mixture.

3. Bake the salmon for 12•15 minutes, or until it flakes easily with a fork.

4. While the salmon is baking, prepare the quinoa salad. In a medium bowl, combine the cooked quinoa, cucumber, tomatoes, parsley, dill, lemon juice, and olive oil. Season with salt and pepper.

5. Serve the baked salmon fillets warm, topped with the lemon herb quinoa salad.

This dish is supportive for a fatty liver diet as it is:
• High in lean protein from the salmon
• Rich in fiber and antioxidants from the quinoa, vegetables, and herbs
• Contains healthy fats from the olive oil
• Uses minimal added sugars or unhealthy ingredients

101. Spinach and feta stuffed portobello mushrooms

Ingredients:
- 4 large portobello mushroom caps, stems removed and chopped
- 2 cups fresh spinach, chopped
- 1/2 cup crumbled feta cheese
- 2 cloves garlic, minced
- 1 tbsp olive oil
- 1/4 tsp dried oregano
- Salt and pepper to taste

Instructions:

1. Preheat the oven to 400°F. Lightly grease a baking sheet or line it with parchment paper.

2. Gently clean the portobello mushroom caps with a damp paper towel. Remove the stems and chop them.

3. In a skillet over medium heat, sauté the chopped mushroom stems and garlic in the olive oil for 2•3 minutes until fragrant.

4. Add the chopped spinach and continue cooking for 2•3 minutes until the spinach is wilted.

5. Remove the skillet from heat and stir in the crumbled feta cheese, oregano, salt, and pepper.

6. Spoon the spinach and feta mixture evenly into the portobello mushroom caps, packing it in gently.

7. Place the stuffed mushrooms on the prepared baking sheet.

8. Bake for 15•20 minutes, until the mushrooms are tender and the filling is hot.

9. Serve the stuffed portobello mushrooms warm.

This dish is supportive for a fatty liver diet as it is:
- High in fiber and antioxidants from the portobello mushrooms and spinach
- Contains healthy fats from the olive oil and feta cheese
- Uses whole food ingredients without added sugars or unhealthy fats

102. Grilled shrimp with mango avocado salsa and quinoa

Ingredients:

Grilled Shrimp:
• 1 lb large shrimp, peeled and deveined
• 2 tbsp olive oil
• 1 tsp chili powder
• 1 tsp garlic powder
• Salt and pepper to taste

Mango Avocado Salsa:
• 1 ripe mango, diced
• 1 avocado, diced
• 1/2 red onion, diced
• 1 jalapeño, seeded and minced
• 1/4 cup chopped cilantro
• 2 tbsp lime juice
• 1 tbsp olive oil
• Salt and pepper to taste

Quinoa:• 1 cup cooked quinoa

Instructions:

1. Preheat grill or grill pan to medium•high heat.

2. In a bowl, toss the shrimp with the olive oil, chili powder, garlic powder, salt, and pepper.

3. Grill the shrimp for 2•3 minutes per side, until opaque and cooked through. Set aside.

4. In a separate bowl, combine all the mango avocado salsa ingredients and mix well. Season with salt and pepper.

5. Serve the grilled shrimp over a bed of cooked quinoa, topped with the mango avocado salsa.

This dish is supportive for a fatty liver diet as it is:
• High in lean protein from the shrimp
• Rich in fiber and antioxidants from the quinoa, mango, avocado, and vegetables
• Contains healthy fats from the olive oil and avocado
• Uses minimal added sugars or unhealthy ingredients

103. Lentil and vegetable soup with whole wheat bread

Ingredients:
- 1 cup brown or green lentils, rinsed
- 4 cups low•sodium vegetable broth
- 1 onion, diced
- 3 carrots, peeled and diced
- 2 celery stalks, diced
- 3 garlic cloves, minced
- 1 tsp ground cumin
- 1 tsp dried oregano
- Salt and pepper to taste
- Chopped parsley for garnish

Instructions:
1. In a large pot, combine the lentils and vegetable broth. Bring to a boil.
2. Reduce heat and simmer for 15•20 minutes, until lentils are tender.
3. Add the onion, carrots, celery, and garlic. Simmer for 10•15 more minutes.
4. Stir in the cumin, oregano, salt, and pepper.
5. Serve hot, garnished with chopped parsley.

Whole Wheat Bread
Ingredients:
- 2 cups whole wheat flour
- 1 tsp baking powder
- 1/2 tsp salt
- 1 cup low•fat milk
- 2 tbsp honey

Instructions:
1. Preheat oven to 375°F. Grease a 9x5 inch loaf pan.
2. In a large bowl, whisk together the whole wheat flour, baking powder, and salt.
3. In a separate bowl, whisk together the milk and honey.
4. Pour the milk mixture into the flour mixture and stir just until combined (do not overmix).
5. Pour the batter into the prepared loaf pan.
6. Bake for 30•35 minutes, until a toothpick inserted in the center comes out clean.
7. Allow to cool for 10 minutes before slicing.

This meal provides a good balance of fiber, protein, and complex carbs from the lentils and whole wheat bread, which can help support a fatty liver diet for women. The vegetables also provide important nutrients.

104. Turkey and vegetable stir fry with brown rice noodles

Ingredients:

- 8 oz brown rice noodles
- 1 lb ground turkey
- 2 tbsp low-sodium soy sauce
- 1 tbsp rice vinegar
- 1 tsp sesame oil
- 1 tbsp grated fresh ginger
- 2 garlic cloves, minced
- 1 red bell pepper, sliced
- 1 cup broccoli florets
- 1 cup sliced mushrooms
- 2 cups baby spinach
- 2 tbsp chopped green onions
- Salt and pepper to taste

Instructions:

1. Cook the brown rice noodles according to package instructions. Drain and set aside.

2. In a large skillet or wok, cook the ground turkey over medium-high heat, breaking it up as it cooks, until no longer pink, about 5-7 minutes. Drain any excess fat.

3. Add the soy sauce, rice vinegar, sesame oil, ginger, and garlic to the skillet. Stir to combine.

4. Add the bell pepper, broccoli, and mushrooms. Stir-fry for 3-4 minutes until vegetables are tender-crisp.

5. Add the cooked noodles and spinach to the skillet. Toss everything together until the spinach is wilted, about 1-2 minutes.

6. Remove from heat and stir in the green onions. Season with salt and pepper to taste.

7. Serve the stir-fry immediately.

This dish is a great option for a fatty liver diet for women. The turkey provides lean protein, the vegetables offer fiber and antioxidants, and the brown rice noodles are a whole grain carb source. The soy sauce, vinegar, and sesame oil add flavor without too much sodium or fat.

105. Quinoa and black bean stuffed bell peppers

Ingredients:

• 4 medium bell peppers, halved lengthwise and seeds removed
• 1 cup cooked quinoa
• 1 (15 oz) can black beans, rinsed and drained
• 1 cup diced tomatoes
• 1/2 cup diced onion
• 2 cloves garlic, minced
• 1 tsp ground cumin
• 1 tsp chili powder
• 1/4 cup chopped fresh cilantro
• Salt and pepper to taste
• 1/2 cup shredded low•fat cheddar cheese (optional)

Instructions:

1. Preheat oven to 375°F. Place the bell pepper halves in a baking dish and set aside.

2. In a medium bowl, combine the cooked quinoa, black beans, diced tomatoes, onion, garlic, cumin, chili powder, and cilantro. Season with salt and pepper.

3. Spoon the quinoa and black bean mixture evenly into the bell pepper halves.

4. If using, sprinkle the shredded cheese over the top of the stuffed peppers.

5. Bake for 25•30 minutes, until the peppers are tender and the filling is hot.

6. Serve the stuffed peppers warm.

This dish is an excellent choice for a fatty liver diet for women. Quinoa is a high•fiber, high•protein grain that is gentle on the liver. Black beans provide additional fiber and plant•based protein. The bell peppers are a great source of vitamins A and C, as well as antioxidants. The dish is low in saturated fat and sodium, making it a healthy and delicious option.

106. Baked cod with roasted vegetables and quinoa

Ingredients:

- 4 (6 oz) cod fillets
- 2 tbsp olive oil, divided
- 1 tsp paprika
- Salt and pepper to taste
- 2 cups cubed butternut squash
- 1 cup Brussels sprouts, halved
- 1 red onion, sliced
- 1 cup cooked quinoa

For the Lemon Herb Sauce:
- 2 tbsp lemon juice
- 1 tbsp chopped fresh parsley
- 1 tbsp chopped fresh dill
- 1 garlic clove, minced
- 2 tbsp low·fat Greek yogurt
- Salt and pepper to taste

Instructions:

1. Preheat oven to 400°F. Line a baking sheet with parchment paper.

2. Place the cod fillets on the prepared baking sheet. Drizzle with 1 tbsp olive oil and sprinkle with paprika, salt, and pepper.

3. In a large bowl, toss the butternut squash, Brussels sprouts, and red onion with the remaining 1 tbsp olive oil. Season with salt and pepper.

4. Spread the vegetables in a single layer on the baking sheet alongside the cod.

5. Bake for 20·25 minutes, until the cod is cooked through and the vegetables are tender.

6. While the cod and vegetables are baking, make the lemon herb sauce. In a small bowl, whisk together the lemon juice, parsley, dill, garlic, and Greek yogurt. Season with salt and pepper.

7. Serve the baked cod over the roasted vegetables and quinoa. Drizzle the lemon herb sauce over the top.

This dish is an excellent choice for a fatty liver diet for women. Cod is a lean, high·protein fish that is gentle on the liver. The roasted vegetables provide fiber, vitamins, and antioxidants. Quinoa is a whole grain that is high in protein and fiber. The lemon herb sauce adds flavor without too much sodium or fat.

107. Lentil and vegetable curry with brown rice

Ingredients:

• 1 cup brown lentils, rinsed
• 4 cups low•sodium vegetable broth
• 1 tbsp olive oil
• 1 onion, diced
• 3 garlic cloves, minced
• 1 tbsp grated fresh ginger
• 2 tsp curry powder
• 1 tsp ground cumin
• 1 tsp ground coriander
• 1 tsp turmeric
• 1 cup diced tomatoes
• 1 cup diced cauliflower
• 1 cup diced sweet potato
• 1 cup frozen peas
• 1/4 cup chopped fresh cilantro
• Salt and pepper to taste
• 2 cups cooked brown rice

Instructions:

1. In a large pot, combine the lentils and vegetable broth. Bring to a boil, then reduce heat and simmer for 15•20 minutes, until lentils are tender.

2. In a large skillet, heat the olive oil over medium heat. Add the onion and sauté for 3•4 minutes until translucent.

3. Add the garlic, ginger, curry powder, cumin, coriander, and turmeric. Stir and cook for 1 minute until fragrant.

4. Add the diced tomatoes, cauliflower, sweet potato, and peas. Stir to combine. Stir the cooked lentils into the vegetable mixture. Simmer for 10•15 minutes, until vegetables are tender.

5. Remove from heat and stir in the chopped cilantro. Season with salt and pepper to taste.. Serve the lentil and vegetable curry over the cooked brown rice.

This dish is an excellent choice for a fatty liver diet for women. Lentils are a great source of plant•based protein and fiber, which can help support liver health. The vegetables provide important vitamins, minerals, and antioxidants. Brown rice is a whole grain that is gentle on the liver.

108. Grilled chicken with steamed broccoli and quinoa

Ingredients:

- 4 (6 oz) boneless, skinless chicken breasts
- 1 tbsp olive oil
- 1 tsp garlic powder
- 1 tsp dried oregano
- Salt and pepper to taste
- 4 cups broccoli florets
- 1 cup cooked quinoa

For the Lemon Herb Sauce:
- 2 tbsp lemon juice
- 1 tbsp chopped fresh parsley
- 1 tbsp chopped fresh basil
- 1 garlic clove, minced
- 1 tbsp olive oil
- Salt and pepper to taste

Instructions:

1. Preheat grill or grill pan to medium•high heat.

2. Rub the chicken breasts with the 1 tbsp olive oil and season with the garlic powder, oregano, salt, and pepper.

3. Grill the chicken for 5•7 minutes per side, or until cooked through. Set aside.

4. Steam the broccoli florets until tender•crisp, about 5•7 minutes.

5. In a small bowl, whisk together the lemon juice, parsley, basil, garlic, 1 tbsp olive oil, salt, and pepper to make the lemon herb sauce.

6. Slice the grilled chicken and serve over the steamed broccoli and cooked quinoa. Drizzle the lemon herb sauce over the top.

This dish is an excellent choice for a fatty liver diet for women. Grilled chicken is a lean protein that is gentle on the liver. Broccoli is a cruciferous vegetable that provides fiber, vitamins, and antioxidants. Quinoa is a whole grain that is high in protein and fiber. The lemon herb sauce adds flavor without too much sodium or fat.

109. Tofu and vegetable stir fry with brown rice

Ingredients:
- 1 cup uncooked brown rice
- 1 block (14 oz) extra•firm tofu, cubed
- 2 tbsp low•sodium soy sauce
- 1 tbsp rice vinegar
- 1 tsp sesame oil
- 1 tbsp grated fresh ginger
- 2 garlic cloves, minced
- 2 cups broccoli florets
- 1 red bell pepper, sliced
- 1 cup sliced mushrooms
- 1 cup snow peas
- 2 green onions, sliced
- 1 tbsp sesame seeds (optional)

Instructions:

1. Cook the brown rice according to package instructions. Set aside.

2. In a medium bowl, combine the cubed tofu, soy sauce, rice vinegar, and sesame oil. Toss to coat the tofu and set aside.

3. Heat a large skillet or wok over medium•high heat. Add the ginger and garlic and cook for 1 minute until fragrant.

4. Add the broccoli, bell pepper, mushrooms, and snow peas. Stir•fry for 5•7 minutes until vegetables are tender•crisp.

5. Add the marinated tofu and its sauce to the skillet. Stir•fry for 2•3 minutes until the tofu is heated through.

6. Remove from heat and stir in the sliced green onions.

7. Serve the tofu and vegetable stir•fry over the cooked brown rice. Sprinkle with sesame seeds if desired.

This dish is an excellent choice for a fatty liver diet for women. Tofu is a plant•based protein that is gentle on the liver. The vegetables provide fiber, vitamins, and antioxidants. Brown rice is a whole grain that is high in fiber and low in fat. The soy sauce, vinegar, and sesame oil add flavor without too much sodium or fat.

110. Turkey and black bean lettuce wraps with a side of quinoa

Ingredients:

- 1 lb ground turkey
- 1 (15 oz) can black beans, rinsed and drained
- 1 cup diced tomatoes
- 1/2 cup diced onion
- 2 garlic cloves, minced
- 1 tsp chili powder
- 1 tsp ground cumin
- Salt and pepper to taste
- 12 large lettuce leaves (such as romaine or bibb)
- 1 cup cooked quinoa

For the Avocado Crema:
- 1 avocado, pitted and mashed
- 2 tbsp plain Greek yogurt
- 1 tbsp lime juice
- 1 tbsp chopped cilantro
- Salt and pepper to taste

Instructions:

1. In a large skillet over medium heat, cook the ground turkey, breaking it up as it cooks, until no longer pink, about 5•7 minutes. Drain any excess fat.

2. Add the black beans, diced tomatoes, onion, garlic, chili powder, and cumin to the skillet. Stir to combine and cook for 2•3 minutes until heated through. Season with salt and pepper.

3. In a small bowl, mash the avocado. Stir in the Greek yogurt, lime juice, and cilantro. Season the avocado crema with salt and pepper.

4. To assemble, place a spoonful of the turkey and black bean mixture into a lettuce leaf. Top with a dollop of the avocado crema. Serve the lettuce wraps with a side of cooked quinoa.

This dish is an excellent choice for a fatty liver diet for women. Ground turkey is a lean protein that is gentle on the liver. Black beans provide fiber and plant•based protein. The lettuce leaves are a low•calorie, nutrient•dense wrap option. Quinoa is a whole grain that is high in fiber and protein. The avocado crema adds healthy fats and creaminess without too much saturated fat.

As we come to the end of ***"Fatty Liver Diet Cookbook for Women: 110+ Wholesome Meals to Nurture Your Liver and Well-being,"*** I hope you have found this book to be an invaluable resource in your journey toward better liver health and overall well-being. This cookbook is more than a collection of recipes; it is a testament to the power of nutritious food in transforming our health and lives.

Celebrating Your Journey

Managing and reversing fatty liver disease is not an overnight process; it is a journey that requires commitment, patience, and self-care. By incorporating the wholesome meals and nutritional principles outlined in this book, you have taken significant steps toward nurturing your liver and enhancing your health. Celebrate your progress, no matter how small, and recognize the positive changes you are making for yourself and your loved ones.

Continued Commitment to Health

The recipes and tips provided in this book are designed to be a sustainable part of your daily life. Continue to explore new flavors, experiment with different ingredients, and make mindful choices that support your liver health. Remember, the foundation of a healthy lifestyle is consistency. By maintaining the dietary and lifestyle changes you have embraced, you can enjoy long-term benefits and a renewed sense of vitality.

Beyond the Kitchen

While this cookbook focuses on nutrition, it is important to acknowledge the holistic nature of health. Regular physical activity, adequate sleep, stress management, and staying hydrated are all crucial components of a healthy lifestyle. Strive to create a balanced and fulfilling life that supports your physical, mental, and emotional well-being.

A Final Note of Gratitude

Thank you for choosing to embark on this journey with "Fatty Liver Diet Cookbook for Women." Your dedication to improving your liver health and well-being is commendable. I am grateful to have been a part of your journey and hope that the recipes and insights shared in this book have empowered you to take control of your health.

Looking Forward

As you continue on your path to better health, remember that every small step counts. Keep exploring, learning, and evolving. Your liver and your body are remarkable, and with the right care, they can thrive. Here's to a healthier, happier you, filled with energy, joy, and the delicious flavors of life.